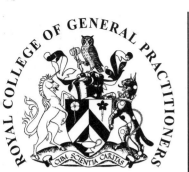

OCCASIONAL PAPER **86**

Getting it right in the consultation: *Hippocrates' problem; Aristotle's answer*

Dr John CM Gillies MA, FRCGP, FRCPEd

Published by
The Royal College of General Practitioners

August 2005

Charter

The Royal College of General Practitioners was founded in 1952, with this object:

To encourage, foster, and maintain the highest possible standards in general medical practice and for that purpose to take or join with others in taking steps consistent with the charitable nature of that object which may assist towards the same.

Among its responsibilities under its Royal Charter the College is entitled to:

Encourage the publication by general medical practitioners of research into medical or scientific subjects with a view to the improvement of general medical practice in any field and to undertake or assist others in undertaking such research.

Diffuse information on all matters affecting general medical practice and establish, print, publish, issue and circulate such papers, journals, magazines, books, periodicals, and publications and hold such meetings, conferences, seminars, and instructional courses as may assist the object of the College.

British Library Cataloguing-in-Publication Data
A catalogue record for this book is available from the British Library.

College Headquarters

The Headquarters of the Royal College is at 14 Princes Gate, Hyde Park, London SW7 1PU (Telephone: 020 7581 3232). Publishing enquiries should be addressed to the Publishing Manager and general enquiries to the Chief Executive.

Occasional Papers

The *Occasional Paper* series was established in 1976 to offer authors the opportunity to publish manuscripts too long for publication as articles and too short for books. They are assessed for academic acceptability by the Editor, College Publications and other professionals with special interests. Readers should note that they express the views of the authors, and not the College, unless otherwise stated.

Occasional papers are included in *Index Medicus*.

Copyright

All rights reserved. No part of this publication may be reproduced, stored in a retrieval system, or transmitted, in any form or by any means, electronic, mechanical, photocopying, recording or otherwise without the prior permission of the Royal College of General Practitioners.

© Royal College of General Practitioners, 2005

Gu mo mhàthair 's gu m'athair – to my mother and father

Contents

Foreword 1

Glossary of terms 2

Introduction 3

Chapter one 5

Hippocrates' problem: decision making in general practice

Chapter two 11

Aristotle's answer (1): a practical reasoning approach

Chapter three 19

Aristotle's answer (2): Decision making in general practice: the practice of perception

Appendix one 28

Appendix two 29

Appendix three 30

Appendix four 31

Appendix five 32

References 34

Foreword

This Occasional Paper adds a new dimension to the theoretical basis of good general practice and complements the work of Toon, Marinker, McWhinney, and others, at a time of rapid change in helping to define what is the distinctive nature of our discipline. The paper covers philosophical works and recent literature concerning the decision-making process in relation to the many and varied complex human interactions that take place in the general practice consultation. This paper is a watershed in thinking at a time of further proposed modernisation in primary care and the importance of the general practitioner as a personal doctor: ensuring continuity of care, acting as the patient's advocate, as well as the gatekeeper in an NHS that is being restructured.

Dr Rodger Charlton MD, FRCGP, FRNZCGP

Glossary of Terms

Aisthesis: perception, capacity to understand particular situations

Autonomy: self-rule – to act autonomously is to act under one's own direction, to be in control of oneself and to be able to make reasonable decisions about what actions to take

Beneficence: the principle of helping others by taking actions that promote the good of others

Consequentialism: the idea that the value of a course of action derives completely from the consequences of that action. (Also see Utilitarianism, below)

Deontology: the view that the correct course of action is based on duties rather than consequences (see above)

Empiricism: the concept that all knowledge is derived from experience, which is ultimately acquired through the senses

Ethics: the study of the concepts involved in practical reasoning: good, right, duty, obligation, virtue, freedom, choice

Hermeneutics: the study of interpretation of texts, also of social, historical and psychological phenomena

Holistic: describing the view that the whole is more than the sum of its parts, when these parts are looked at individually – often contrasted with reductionism (see below)

Incommensurable: not able to be compared by applying a single measure

Non-maleficence: obeying this principle means a duty not to inflict harm on others – in medical ethics, it is illustrated by the aphorism: *primum non nocere* (first of all, do no harm)

Normative: prescriptive, applying a norm or standard

Organismic: based on the idea that responses are those of a living being or organism, rather than an abstract idea of an organ or system

Paradigm: a framework of concepts, results and procedures within which subsequent work is structured and understood

Paternalism: the principle of intentionally interfering with someone's life to achieve good, or to avoid harm coming to him or her

Phantasia: the capability of focusing on a concrete particular, past or absent, and discerning its content

Phronesis: practical wisdom, the ability to decide correctly what to do in practical situations

Reductionism: the idea that complex phenomena can be understood fully by reducing them to fewer or simpler phenomena or facts

Reification: treating a concept as if it automatically refers to a thing with external reality

Teleological: refers to the concept that life has an end or purpose

Utilitarianism: the group of ethical theories that hold that what is important is to achieve the greatest good for the greatest number – all utilitarian theories are therefore consequentialist (see above)

Virtue ethics: based on the idea that it is the virtues of the good person that are of prime importance in determining what is the appropriate course of action in any situation, rather than duties (see deontology) or consequences (see consequentialism and utilitarianism)

Terms in italics are Ancient Greek words. Many of these definitions come from: Blackburn S. *A Dictionary of Philosophy*, Oxford: Oxford University Press, 1994, and Beauchamp T, and Childress J. *Principles of Medical Ethics* (5th Edition) Oxford, Oxford University Press, 2001.

Terms that are included here in the glossary are shown in bold throughout the text.

Introduction

I wrote this paper as a result of my concerns about some current trends in general practice in the UK today. Medicine in general has become much more evidence based, and general practice has followed this trend. It is the most important step forward in my professional lifetime as a GP, and it can both improve quality of care in general practice and save many patients' lives. My concerns stem from what I see as a tendency to believe that the *evidence*, which is always population based and general, can be simply applied to the *practice* of our discipline with individual patients. The former is based firmly on **empiricism**; the latter, I suggest, should use empirical evidence, but should not necessarily privilege it over other important considerations closer to the patient. This is not just a philosophical or theoretical worry; applications of evidence, if poorly thought out, can cost as well as save lives. When the basis of our new GMS (General Medical Services) contract is evidence, we need to consider these matters seriously. In the future of general practice, whatever that may be, I think that it is important that *scientia* and *caritas,* the two elements of the motto of the RCGP, are both held to be valuable. This paper provides an argument for this position.

I am also well aware that there are approaches to this issue based on complexity theory rather than philosophy.[1–3] These are a welcome addition to the literature on general practice, and are helping to shift our collective professional mindset. It is reasonable to ask therefore, why we need to go back through more than two thousand years of philosophy, as in this paper, rather than thirty years of new theoretical approaches, to look for answers. Answering that question might need another paper. Briefly, my response is that although science has transformed our lives over the past century, human nature has probably not changed over two millennia, and we ignore that accumulated wisdom, reflected in philosophical writing, at our peril. It still has much to tell us. Modern philosophers of the Greek world often suggest, ironically, that the Ancients keep stealing our ideas. Behind much current work on complexity and general practice, I believe, lies the sort of practical reasoning that I describe in this paper.

Hippocrates' Problem

Hippocrates' problem is that of making decisions with patients in general practice. This is the context of a discipline which is, according to one prominent general practitioner (GP) 'blurry at the edges'.[i] GPs look after individuals, families and their communities. There is a shortage of empirical evidence for much of the work of general practice. As society changes, so must the content and practice of the discipline. General practice has evolved from a demoralised, overburdened discipline in the 1950s to one with a growing academic status and reputation.

Chapter One

Hippocrates' problem: decision making in general practice

The breadth and 'blurriness' of the discipline of general practice outlined above obviously make it difficult to fit into a standard scientific model. The biomedical model, the anticipatory care model and teleological/hermeneutic models[4] are briefly discussed in chapter one. I also discuss some recent work on evidence based and narrative based medicine and the ideas of McWhinney. His analysis of general practice[5] is that of a relationship based discipline, focused on individual patients, based on an **organismic** rather than a mechanistic metaphor, and transcending the mind–body division on which modern medicine has been founded. I suggest that this offers a rounded picture of the discipline that acknowledges its 'blurriness', and, perhaps for the first time, gives a definitive perspective that is qualitatively very different from other models. Decisions with patients should acknowledge the inherent complexities of this analysis.

Chapter Two

Aristotle's answer (1): a practical reasoning approach

How do we make good decisions with our patients? This question illustrates the general problem of choosing correctly, which has exercised philosophers over more than two millennia. The dominant **normative** ethical theories of our time that address this problem are based either on **consequentialism** or on **deontology**.

Consequentialism is the view that the right action in a situation should be based on the value of the results or consequences of that action. **Utilitarianism**, which is based on maximising the good, is a consequentialist concept. Deontological theories, in contrast, are founded on the view that correct actions should be based on our duties, and whether an action is right or wrong is determined by the action itself, not by its consequences. These theoretical approaches represent what David Raphael[ii] describes as 'two different and stubbornly persistent outlooks on **ethics**'.

A major problem with these two theories is that neither can rule out the possibility of major disagreements that cannot be resolved.[6, p.210] Both types of normative theory, Wiggins[6] suggests, attempt to rule out the possibility of such disagreements by stating in advance what counts in making decisions, and what does not.

This inability to completely resolve disagreements is a fundamental problem. In practical situations, we can see the implications of this. If we are trying to decide what to do in consultations with patients in general practice, with its inherent complexities and mix of clinical, public health and social problems, looking to normative ethical theories to tell us what to do is particularly beset by difficulties,

---

i   This phrase comes from a lecture in 1998 delivered at Dunkeld by Dr Graham Buckley, then Chief Executive, NHS Education Scotland.
ii This statement comes from course notes circulated by Professor Raphael at the Imperial College Medical Ethics course, 11–15th September 2000.

as areas of conflict and disagreement arise continually. If these cannot be resolved by recourse to a theoretical position, what then is the way forward?

Rather than seeking to eliminate disagreement through formulating normative theories, Wiggins[6] believes that we should seek agreement through 'the familiar processes of reasoning, conversion and criticism' but do so in the knowledge that we will never be *wholly* successful in achieving agreement by these means.

The way forward, therefore, may be to lay ethical theory to one side (but not to reject either duties or consequences out of hand, nor to suggest that they are of no relevance), and to consider a very different approach. *This is the basis of Aristotle's answer to Hippocrates' problem.*

Aristotle suggests that we focus on each individual case, each particular situation. The approach described is derived both from Aristotle directly, and from recent papers by philosophers who are widely recognised as major figures in Aristotelian scholarship, namely Wiggins,[6,10] McDowell,[7] and Nussbaum.[8]

It is based on what McDowell[7, p.51] calls a 'perceptual capacity'. This is central to his conception of the virtuous agent, and is a form of knowledge of how to behave in particular situations, a 'sensitivity to a certain sort of requirement that situations impose on behaviour'.

The account that I set out will include a discussion of what Nussbaum[8, p.155] calls 'the priority of the particular', and an exploration of 'perceptual capacity', which will include a discussion of the importance of imagination and the emotions in correct choosing.

Chapter Three

Aristotle's answer (2): the practice of perception

The practice of perception refers to the way in which the practical reasoning approach may be pertinent in general practice. I will relate McWhinney's conception of general practice to the practical reasoning approach. McWhinney's focus on the particulars of the consultation is reflected in the priority of the particular. This offers an understanding of different facets of clinical particularity – indeterminacy, novel clinical problems and approaches, and the uniqueness of the encounter.

The central problem of decision making in general practice is the need 'to sort the unsorted'.[9, p.39] The position that I set out is one that requires an approach that is focused on the particular situation, and applies to it a well-developed 'perceptual capacity' or 'situational appreciation'.[10, p.237] This requires imagination and the appropriate degree of emotional involvement.

Clinical encounters in practice are often irreducibly complex. Evidence, in the form of rules or clinical guidelines, needs to be considered and adapted to the situation rather than be used to pre-determine the outcome of the encounter. Principles[11, chs. 3–6] are likewise considered in the light of the situation, rather than as providing an over-arching framework. Dealing with a clinical situation requires judgement, born of experience and careful training, and informed by deliberation on all the relevant circumstances impinging on that situation. The description of intuition by Greenhalgh[12] contains many elements of the practice of perception. The assessment of video tapes of consultations for summative assessment and the RCGP examination is firmly based on perceptual capacity. There is also a developing literature on relational empathy, which is also strongly related to perceptual capacity. The new GMS contract for GPs, however, is at heart a utilitarian document and privileges evidence over perception. In this chapter, I look at some ways in which this issue might be addressed.

The over-riding aim of the practice of perception is to achieve what is best for *the patient in that situation*. However, the outcome is always determined by the practicalities of the context. I illustrate this with an example: Dr Lawrence's problem, set out in Appendix one.

Acknowledgements

It is a cliché to say that our patients are our greatest teachers, but this was never more true than of this paper. I also owe a great debt to my training practice, in particular Dr David Strachan and the late Drs Connie Gibb and Alastair Donald. My GP partners, past and present, and many professional colleagues and friends have stimulated, challenged and broadened my thinking. Nurses can sometimes be more perceptive than doctors, and working with Sister Margaret Young and her staff at Selkirk has made me very aware of this. Dr Peter Toon's Occasional Papers stimulated my initial interest in the area. Professor Kenneth Boyd taught me how to find out about philosophy and medical ethics. The teaching staff at the Centre for Professional Ethics at Keele University provided a learning environment that was supportive, challenging and stimulating. In particular, I am grateful to Dr Mark P Sheehan for many discussions and arguments. Dr Andrew Riley, Director of Public Health, NHS Borders, generously supported me through a postgraduate course that had as much to do with general practice as public health. Drs Iain Bamforth, Bill Currie, Mary Low, and the late Janet Heyes provided invaluable comments and criticism. My understanding of the use of instruments to assess what happens in the consultation has been considerably improved by discussions with Professor John Howie and Dr Stewart Mercer. My thanks to Ruth O'Rourke and Helen Farrelly of RCGP Publications for their careful editing and helpful suggestions. Dr Patrick Manson suggested that good consultations are characterised by 'getting it right'. To my wife, Dr Mary Gillies, I owe a triple debt, for many useful critical comments, for proof reading, and for the opportunity cost of many weekends spent at the keyboard. Any mistakes remain my own.

Chapter One
Hippocrates' Problem: Decision Making in General Practice

General practice 'is accepted as being something specific, without anyone knowing what it really is'. Collings [13, p.555]

Introduction

Hippocrates' problem is that of making decisions with patients. Here is an example:

Margaret Smith is a 79-year-old woman with a recent diagnosis of breast cancer. She lives alone in poor social circumstances, has little family support and also has other health problems. She has had a mastectomy, but despite the advice of the oncologist treating her, she is not currently keen to have either radiotherapy or chemotherapy, and says that she wants to 'take her chances'. Her longstanding GP, Dr Lawrence sees her regularly. He has to advise her, and help her to decide what to do.

This example illustrates the mix of physical, psychological and social factors that make up general practice, a discipline where the facts don't always tell you what to do. A more detailed discussion of this case can be found in appendix one on page 28. This paper will set out an approach to such problems based on Aristotle's ethics.

To understand decision-making in general practice and how it might best be carried out, I will discuss the definition of the nature of general practice, and the qualities, competencies and abilities required by the general practitioner. This chapter will review some of the literature on this and examine current ideas on the subject. Some historical detail will help to put the current situation in perspective. Although this section contains little philosophical analysis, it will give background on the subject, which will put the practical reasoning approach into context.

General practice is a craft or branch of medicine. It embraces all the activities of doctors who are the first point of contact for a patient 'who is ill, or who believes himself to be ill'.[14, pp.273-74] We are often the doctors of both first and last resort for our patients.

The Past Fifty Years

A visit to a general practitioner is familiar to almost everyone. In the UK, a GP will see two thirds of his patients in one year, and ninety per cent over five years.[15, p.407] GPs assess, diagnose and treat their patients. The GP also acts as gatekeeper to the skills or opinions of specialists who work in hospitals.

Lord Moran, Winston Churchill's physician, described general practitioners in 1966 as those who had fallen from the ladder of advancement.[16, p.84] This condescending view was perhaps marginally less insulting than the description by Sir Clifford Allbutt in a letter to the Times in 1912 of general practice as, 'very perfunctory work, (which) fell into the hands of perfunctory men'.[16, p.55] Both men were Presidents of the Royal College of Physicians of London. These views were widely shared by many hospital doctors.

After the founding of the NHS in 1948, each GP became contractually responsible for the medical care of patients on his or her list twenty-four hours a day, seven days a week. List size varied between two and four thousand patients. Group practice at the time was very rare, and GPs competed for patients, as income was largely a function of number of patients served, rather than services provided. Consultations were short, visiting rates very high, and night work an inescapable part of the job. Workload in areas of deprivation (which were many after the Second World War) was especially gruelling. There was no general practice specific training, and many graduates entered practice directly after one year's hospital experience.

These huge pressures on general practice, which reflected a society adapting to an NHS free at the point of delivery of care, and a population with high rates of cancer, heart disease, tuberculosis and other infectious diseases, are well described in Collings' account. He describes a morning in a city practice in 1949 thus:

During my stay of an hour and a quarter about one hundred and twenty patients came in. They were 'seen' by three different doctors, who replaced one another with almost bewildering rapidity. No pretence was made at real examination of any of these patients. An occasional temperature or pulse rate was taken; four or five times a stethoscope was applied to a point somewhere below the thyroid gland and some such utterance made as 'ah, a bit chesty'.[13, p.563]

While the medicine may perforce have been perfunctory, the men (and they were nearly all men) often were not. Collings describes many examples of GPs attempting to provide medical care of high quality under extremely difficult conditions. This is his description of such a practice:

All patients were seen by appointment; a quarter of an hour was assigned to each, but whenever necessary more time was given. Patients on return visits requiring certificates or repeat prescriptions were asked to come at the beginning of the consulting hour, and ten to twelve came within the hour. Physical examinations were thorough and reasonably full records were kept. During my time in this practice I saw no-one referred for an opinion until the case had been investigated as far as possible in the surgery.[13, p.564]

While many GPs adjusted their standards downward to cope with the overwhelming demands of their patients, others made a determined effort to provide quality of care and professional satisfaction.

The following sections discuss some aspects of the development of general practice over the past fifty years.

Balint

Balint's seminal work *The Doctor, his Patient and the Illness* published in 1964, was the first to consider, in psychoanalytical terms, the nature of the doctor–patient relationship in general practice.[17] There were two aspects to the thinking of the Balint group of doctors. One was that the illness was perceived as part of the person, not as an externalised phenomenon, an example of a disease process. The other was that of 'the drug doctor', the phrase developed to describe the therapeutic effect of the doctor, mediated through the doctor–patient relationship.

Although neither of these concepts was new, their articulation and publication at this time by a group of individuals who subsequently became prominent in the shaping of general practice in the UK, marked the beginning of a shift away from the purely biomechanical model of medical practice, which was the prevailing one at the time. The consequences were considerable; one major effect was to allow or encourage the GP to concentrate on the circumstances of the individual patient before him, rather than view the patient as an example of a disease.

This of course means that treatment has to be individualised *to that situation,* and has considerable implications for the way in which judgements and decisions are made by the GP. If decisions are to be based on the particular circumstances of the individual, then an approach that reflects this needs to be elaborated. This focus on the individual is reflected in the 'priority of the particular',[8, p.155] an important aspect of Aristotle's answer, the practical reasoning approach.

The Good Doctor

In a paper entitled *What sort of doctor?*,[18] a working group of the RCGP considered values in general practice. They listed the following:

Nine value statements

- The doctor tries to render a personal service which is comprehensive and continuing.
- In his practice arrangements he balances his own convenience against that of his patients, takes into account his responsibility to the wider practice community, and is mindful of the interests of society at large.
- He accepts the obligation to maintain his own mental and physical health.
- He puts a high value on communication skills.
- He subjects his work to critical self-scrutiny and peer review, and accepts a commitment to improve his skills and widen his range of services in response to newly disclosed needs.
- He recognises that researching his discipline and teaching others are part of his professional obligations.
- He sees that part of his professional role is to bring about a measure of independence: he encourages self-help and keeps in bounds his own need to be needed.
- His clinical decisions reflect the true long-term interests of his patients.
- He is careful to preserve confidentiality.

This set of values is comprehensive and demanding. Clearly, the discipline of general practice embraces considerable complexity. The good GP has to be not only a reflective scientist with an understanding of research and teaching, but someone who can both listen to his or her patients and impart information in terms that they understand. To provide a personal service, he needs to be available to his or her patients, and to be able to form professional relationships with a wide spectrum of individuals. Good GPs must look after their own health, balance the needs of individual patients and of the community, listen but not tell, and avoid patients becoming dependent on them. These values are reflected, to some extent in the 'Duties and responsibilities of doctors' laid out in the General Medical Council (GMC) publication *Good Medical Practice* published in 2001.[19] However, the GMC document, as the sub-title suggests, is a deontological one, clearly laying out duties, in a form closely approaching that of a book of rules for doctors.

The RCGP document, on the other hand, by approaching the issue from the perspective of personal and professional values rather than rules, suggests that an approach based on **virtue ethics** might be more appropriate than a deontological one for general practice. The practical reasoning approach set out in chapters two and three of this paper is based on the doctor's ability to read a situation correctly, and apply to it his or her accumulated experience and his or her judgement – described by Sheehan as '(a kind of) virtue ethics'.[20]

What is *Good* General Practice?

The epigraph to this chapter suggests that in 1950, little thought had gone into what general practice was, or should be. Forty years of investment of time and energy by groups such as that led by Balint, and by organisations like the RCGP meant that, by the 1990s, general practice was accepted as a craft within medicine, as a suitable career for medical graduates, and as an academic discipline, albeit one with far fewer career academic posts than most long established branches of medicine.[iii]

The public had always valued general practice, it was suggested, and now there was also an understanding that the groundwork of establishing general practice within the medical and academic firmaments had been completed. In parallel with this process, the value statements above provided a professional framework for the aspiring and established general practitioner.

---

iii In 1990, there were only three Chairs of General Practice at four Scottish medical schools, despite the fact that over 50% of medical graduates enter general practice. There are now ten, which suggests some progress.

However, what also became clear was that general practice was in many ways very *unlike* other branches of medicine. Some branches, like surgery and obstetrics, are based largely on the exercise of specialist therapeutic, technical skills. Others, like cardiology or gastroenterology, depend on a detailed knowledge of one aspect of human anatomy and pathophysiology. Still others, like geriatric medicine or paediatrics, relate only to one stage of life. Only general practice embraces all of the above, and many other hard-to-define aspects of disease and illness.[iv]

Balint had, by exploring the relationship between doctor, patient and illness, started to address the challenge inherent in the epigraph to this chapter. His model has powerfully influenced the development of general practice over the past fifty years.

Toon[4] lays out a philosophical analysis of the question, 'What is good general practice?' The issues raised in this paper are of considerable importance in addressing the problem of decision-making in general practice. Except where indicated, the following sections, to page 9, express Toon's views.

The Nature of Good

How does one define good general practice? Toon[4, pp.6–7] suggests that much discussion on this has been based on the collection and analysis of empirical data on different aspects of practice, such as audit data on the care of patients with chronic conditions like diabetes, asthma and hypertension. As we have moved towards care driven by clinical guidelines or protocols, compliance with which is subsequently audited, this way of assessing quality or 'good' general practice has become dominant.[v] This carries the danger of defining the good simply as what is most easily measured in general practice, neatly side-stepping the issue of defining the good.

Different Models

Toon then analyses several models of general practice. Because the focus of this dissertation is on decision making, I will discuss in detail only the biomedical model, the anticipatory care model and the **teleological/ hermeneutic** models. Toon also discusses general practice as a business, and the relationship between the doctor, the patient and the family. These are peripheral to this paper, and will not be further discussed.

Biomedical model – In the biomedical model, the doctor's aim is the diagnosis and management of disease by scientific means. The body is seen as a mechanism, and the doctor mends the broken parts when they break down. Mending can be achieved by drugs, surgery or sometimes replacement of an organ or joint that is broken beyond repair. It is therefore essentially a technical or biomechanical model. The achievements of the model have subsequently been very well described by LeFanu,[25, Chs.1–12] and include the development of penicillin, tuberculosis treatment, hip replacements, intensive care techniques, kidney and heart transplants, drugs for high blood pressure, heart disease and cancer, and infertility treatments.

While this model may provide a very useful approach for the patient who has a life-threatening illness or a disorder amenable to surgical management, it fits general practice less well. Patients presenting to GPs often have ill-defined disorders and feelings of unease, mental or physical discomfort that defy easy categorisation.[9, pp.33–36] Toon gives examples[4, pp.20–21] of how the biomedical approach can usefully be applied to conditions treated in general practice, but points out that for many patients, it is an approach that leads to unhelpful results. Although it may be said to have deontological features in that the doctor has a duty of care to the patient, ultimately, it relies on the consequentialist view 'that life ought to be about longevity and fertility and little else.[4, p.22]

It may also degrade the doctor–patient relationship, as it treats medicine as a technical skill, and ill human beings as machines. It takes no account of distributive justice as it only deals with the needs of individuals one by one, and it treats illness as something detached from the life of the patient. It deals with physical illness of psychological origin, an important part of the spectrum of general practice, with great difficulty, if at all.

In essence, it asserts that the aim of medicine is that of achieving good biological functioning, and ignores the values that the individual human being may attach to such functioning.[vi]

The anticipatory care model – This model is based on the premise that prevention is better than cure. It starts from the view that the illnesses that are major causes of death and disability today have their origins in our behavioural patterns. These include tobacco smoking, excessive alcohol consumption, unhealthy eating or sexual

---

iv Popper[21, p.67] states 'we are students of problems, not of disciplines'. Disciplines in scientific subjects find their form and shape for historical and administrative reasons. However, the need to solve practical problems means that we often have to *cross* disciplinary borders, and avoid our thinking being circumscribed by one discipline. McWhinney[22, p.10] suggests that this accurately describes the nature of addressing problems in general practice.

v Evaluation of health services is increasingly performed through the interpretation of audit data. The production of this data is seen as a method of ensuring both value for money and quality of care. There are many wider points here about the use of audit in medicine and in many areas of society, effectively made by Michael Power.[23] Power's view[pp.10–14] is that the audit process contains paradoxes. The most obvious is that at one level the auditee is not trusted, hence the need for audit, yet at the same time the auditee is trusted to produce reliable audit data. The process of audit itself is regarded as being above criticism. Another point is that not everything can be audited, and the selection of criteria for audit can be a means of effective yet indirect control over the processes of medical care.[23, pp.104–109] The use of waiting list figures to direct the use of health care resources is an obvious example.[24, p.188] The use of audit to fulfil the demands of the nGMS contract is another, which will be discussed further in chapter three. However, within general practice, there is little doubt that clinical and organisational audit, directed by the GP can be a powerful tool, giving the GP useful data on his practice or patients. The key aspect is *how* such data is used in decision making. This is an important aspect of practical reasoning, and is considered in chapters two and three.

vi A further risk of the biomedical approach is medicalisation of every aspect of the human condition, as the pharmaceutical industry increasingly drives medical research. Seventy per cent of funding for drug trials in the USA comes from pharmaceutical firms rather than public sources[26, p.1540] with obvious dangers of bias both in choice of research area and interpretation. The dangers of the creation of new diseases is well illustrated by the recent debate about female sexual dysfunction.[27, p.45] An emphasis on the biological aspects of this condition, and a downplaying of important relationship, psychological and socio–cultural factors is apparent, driven by the development of new drugs.

practices, as well as the complex effects of deprivation on behaviour. The function of the doctor is to prevent the onset of these diseases by undertaking preventive medicine. This model has been promoted most notably by Julian Tudor Hart. His book *A New Kind of Doctor*[16] provides both the rationale and the methodology for many of these practices.

How does the doctor prevent diseases? Screening, treatment of asymptomatic risk factors, immunisation and health education are the major techniques. The patient list system of general practice produces a database ideal for all these activities. So antenatal care, cervical cytology, childhood immunisations, blood pressure, blood glucose and cholesterol measurement can be easily undertaken. Advice on all sorts of human activity, from sex to diet to exercise can be given either at clinics, or opportunistically.

Like the biomedical model, it is based on the analysis of empirical data on disease epidemiology, and on a mechanical view of the body. However, there is a major philosophical difference between this model and the biomedical and teleological models (see below). The focus of the anticipatory model on maximising health *for a population*, rather than dealing with the problems of individuals, demonstrates a consequentialist approach to health care. The teleological model is essentially deontological, as it is based on the duty of a doctor to an individual patient. The biomedical model has both deontological and consequentialist elements, as discussed on page 7.

In anticipatory care, it can be suggested that autonomy is not properly respected. The health of the patient and the treatment of his or her illness may be considered as means to public health ends such as good cervical screening figures, good population blood pressure control, rather than ends in themselves.[4, p.34] Such a model, in which the doctor rather than the patient sets the agenda, may also be considered paternalistic or authoritarian.

Teleological or hermeneutic models – Teleological models share a conception of life as having an end or purpose. In medicine, that purpose may be achieved by helping the patient to understand or interpret his illness, as well as or instead of the curative role, hence the adjective hermeneutic. They are based on the belief that 'all men by nature reach out for understanding'.[28, p.xv] The Balint movement is used by Toon as an example of such a model. The shift of emphasis from disease to illness is central to this approach. In contrast to the biomedical model, the Balint movement views the illness as part of the individual's life story, and the role of the doctor is that of 'helping the patient to integrate it into a personal life narrative'.[4, p.27] This is a world away from the biomedical model.

A further important point is that in this model, the conventional notion of **autonomy**, based on the concept of interactions between two rational individuals, is rejected. The relationship between doctor and patient is intrinsically an unequal one. Toon[4, p.29] suggests that the personal autonomy of the patient might be sacrificed to a longer-term teleological model of greater autonomy through personal growth enabled by the doctor–patient relationship. Thus, it seems to rely on a **paternalistic** conception of the doctor to achieve the necessary **beneficent** effect.

So What is Good General Practice?

Toon himself admits that his analysis does not lead to a clear answer to this question.[4, p.48] However, he successfully challenges many of the assumptions behind current definitions of what good general practice is, and demonstrates ways in which different models are incompatible both practically and philosophically.[vii]

In summarising,[4, p.48] he makes the important point that patients also use different models when visiting a GP. Some view their bodies as machines that need repair (biomedical model) or servicing (anticipatory care model). Some want to understand why things have gone wrong (teleological/hermeneutic models). Individuals may also switch between models as their illnesses and their understanding of their illnesses evolve.

It is obvious that the consultation and process of care can go badly wrong if the doctor and the patient are using different models. One answer to this problem, addressed in the practical reasoning approach, is that good general practice requires that the doctor is able to *correctly perceive the essential elements of each situation, and hence make the decisions that are most appropriate for that situation*. One of these essential elements is an understanding of what model the patient may currently be using. This sensitivity of approach to a clinical encounter is an important part of what I describe as *the practice of perception*.

Evidence-based and Narrative-based Medicine

Since the publication of Toon's paper in 1994, a considerable amount has been published of relevance to all three models. In particular, the rise of evidence-based medicine (EBM) has helped to clarify the scientific basis of biomedical and anticipatory care. It is described by one of its leading exponents[31, p.71] as:

> *the conscientious, explicit, and judicious use of current best evidence in making decisions about the care of individual patients. The practice of evidence based medicine means integrating individual clinical expertise with the best available external clinical evidence from systematic research.*

EBM, therefore, is concerned with ensuring that the empirical evidence used by doctors and patients is of the highest quality, but allows for its interpretation by the clinician dealing with the individual patient.

---

vii In a further paper in 1999, Toon uses McIntyre's definition of *a practice* as the centrepiece.[29] This is defined as a 'coherent and complex form of socially established co-operative human activity' which realises 'goods internal to that activity' while being rooted in a tradition and contributing to a very Aristotelian conception of human flourishing.[30, pp.187–8] Toon's view[29, pp.43–44] is that practical wisdom is one of several important virtues and does not occupy a central place in defining the virtuous general practitioner. (*The practice of perception*, as defined in this paper is not related to McIntyre's definition.)

Stimulated by the biomedical bias of some exponents of EBM, there have been many recent publications on narrative-based medicine. This focuses on the story that the patient tells, and how both doctor and patient interpret that story. It is therefore hermeneutic in nature, and may be thought of as a development of the Balint model of practice.[32, p.14] Greenhalgh[33, p.257] discusses how evidence is framed and rendered coherent only by the interpreted story of the patient:

In acknowledging the interpretive nature of clinical understanding, we are forced to reject the notion of pure objectivity, for the very existence of interpretive possibilities implies subjectivity, ambiguity and room for disagreement.

This is of course, the world of medicine viewed from the perspective of the individual, rather than the population-based evidence. Yet Sackett's 'individual clinical expertise' is surely related to 'the interpretive nature of clinical understanding'. Both Sackett and Greenhalgh appear to be saying that evidence and narrative approaches are not contradictory but complementary.

The description so far in this chapter of different models of general practice is unsatisfactory, in that none appears to provide a well-rounded model that reflects all aspects of the discipline. The last section will describe an analysis of general practice, which I believe to be a good basis for *the practice of perception*.

The Importance of Being Different

McWhinney[5, pp.433–36] provides a view of general practice that highlights how it differs from other disciplines within medicine. He suggests four main differences:

- It is the only discipline to define itself in terms of relationships, especially the doctor–patient relationship.
- General practitioners tend to think in terms of individual patients, rather than generalised abstractions.
- General practice is based on an **organismic** rather than a mechanistic metaphor of biology.
- General practice is the only major field in medicine that transcends the dualistic division between mind and body.

On the first point, that of relationships, he points out that GPs are not tied to 'diseases, organ systems or technologies'. Their relationship with patients is usually *prior* to the clinical content of the consultation. In other words, they know the characteristics of the individual patient from previous encounters, before the characteristics of the illness or disease become apparent.

The central place of relationships means that GPs are uncomfortable with the biomedical model. In a relationship-based discipline, we will know the world through experience, and therefore through our feelings as well as our intellect, as feelings are an important aspect of experience. This obviously has important consequences for the way in which decisions are made, and a properly rounded approach to decision making will have to include both emotional and intellectual aspects. My claim, outlined in detail in chapters two and three, is that a practical reasoning approach may offer a satisfactory way of addressing this.

On the second point, McWhinney suggests that GPs have difficulty in thinking or talking about diseases without thinking of individual patients who have these diseases. This means a focus on the particular instance, rather than the general or universal. He acknowledges the important gains in medical knowledge that have stemmed from looking at diseases in abstract terms, and suggests that the ideal is an integration of the two views: 'an ability to see the universal in the particular'[5, p.434]. I will suggest that in making judgements in general practice, a focus on the particular is central to making good decisions.

His third point is essentially that human beings cannot be properly understood using a biomedical model. Although the machine-based metaphor can be used to explain some of the simpler features of the working of the human body, the properties of growth, healing, learning and what he describes as 'self-organisation and self-transcendence' are not mechanical. His analysis of the 'multilevel and non-linear' aspects of organismic thinking, with an emphasis on information flows and feedback loops is the basis for the complexity approach to medicine.[viii, 2]

Organismic thinking,[ix] therefore, moving on to the fourth point, makes the mind–body distinction not only untenable but unscientific. The traditions of medicine have led to the division of specialities into those that deal with the body – general medicine, paediatrics, surgery for example, and those that deal with the mind – psychiatry and psychotherapy. McWhinney describes this mind–body division as running through medicine like 'a geological fault'.

General practice, because it deals with undifferentiated illness in individual patients, which may have its primary origin in either mind or body or possibly both, cannot afford the deceptive simplicity of this distinction. The value of the discipline is that of dealing with the whole person – body *and* mind.

He further suggests[5, p.436] 'we can only attend to a patient's feelings and emotions if we know our own'. During the course of the long-term relationships that characterise general practice, emotions arise that doctors must learn to acknowledge and use, both to ensure their own health, and for the therapeutic benefit of their patients. This was one of the great contributions of Balint[17, Chs XIV,XV] to the development of general practice. This awareness can only be achieved, says McWhinney, if we become a 'self-reflective discipline', if we are to be 'healers as well as competent technologists'. This important idea will be further explored in chapter three.

---

viii Foss[34] provides a very detailed analysis of complexity concepts, drawing on empirical and philosophical arguments. He calls the new 'successor' model, which is replacing biomedicine, *info-medicine*.[chs. 23, 24] This describes the multi-level, organism-like features sketched here.

ix The concept of 'organismic thinking' first appears in the writings of Kurt Goldstein, a medical refugee from Nazi Germany, in 1931.[35, pp.145–51] Goldstein thought that medicine in Weimar Germany was becoming overly mechanistic, and sought something that he described as '**holistic rationality.**'

Conclusion

This chapter has given a short overview of changing thinking about general practice over the past few decades. From early post-war days, when GPs struggled to provide basic medical care with few resources and staff, for a war-weary, unhealthy population, it has developed into a discipline with a growing academic literature and status. Toon's discussion exposes many different contradictions of conceptions of good general practice. Nevertheless, we have moved a long way from our initial epigraph to the detailed and thoughtful understanding of general practice provided by McWhinney.

What has become apparent is that many cardinal features of general practice – long-term relationships, the focus on the individual, an organismic view of the human being, and a rejection of mind–body divisions make it a different discipline to any other in medicine. Foss[34, p.257] and McWhinney[5] claim that general practice is in the vanguard of a Kuhnian **paradigm** shift[x] for the whole of medicine. Central to this analysis is the view that the biomedical and anticipatory care models, though important, are offering only part of the overall picture. The recent concentration on the narrative[33] has developed from an awareness of the limitations of this view; what exactly the narrative adds will be explored in chapter three.

McWhinney's 'differences' are reflected in the ways that decisions are made in general practice. The focus on the particular, and the requirement for the GP to respond intellectually and emotionally to the patient are central to both Balint's and McWhinney's analysis. These are the elements of the practical reasoning approach; chapters two and three will attempt to explain why this offers a distinctive and coherent approach to decision making in general practice, and why general practice is fundamentally, *the practice of perception*.

---

x These claims are based on an interpretation of Kuhn.[36, pp.86–89] Kuhn's major claim is that a new paradigm emerges when anomalies within the old paradigm render it unsupportable. However, a new paradigm is likely to contain, or 'enfold' in McWhinney's words, many elements of the old.

Chapter Two
Aristotle's Answer (1): A Practical Reasoning Approach

Man is the measure of all things.
Protagoras the Sophist (c490–c420BC)

Introduction

Discussion about ethics is currently dominated by two theoretical approaches: deontology and consequentialism. Deontological theories are based on the view that correct actions should be based on our duties, and whether an action is right or wrong is determined by the action itself, rather than by its consequences. Such approaches are founded on the work of Immanuel Kant.[37] Consequentialism, on the other hand, is the view that the right action in a situation should be based on the value of the results or consequences of that action.[38]

The approach developed in this chapter is one based not on either category of ethical theory, but on Aristotle's account of practical reasoning. However, I wish first to briefly discuss deontological and consequentialist theories. In the introduction, I touched on one difficulty with such theories and practical decision making. They each take a position on what counts in making decisions – duties for deontological theories and consequences for consequentialist theories. These positions cannot rule out the possibility, as Wiggins[6, p.210] points out, of substantive disagreement, and this may lead to difficulties in practical situations, where duties and consequences may *both* be of importance.

Deontological Theories

Deontological theories are based on the view that correct actions should be based on our duties, and whether an action is right or wrong is determined by the action itself, rather than by its consequences. Such theories suggest that we should look to our over-arching duties, from which are derived rules that should bring clarity to our thinking, and show us what is the right decision to take in any situation. What follows is not a comprehensive review of such theories, merely a brief discussion of some problems associated with rules.

Wittgenstein[39, p.454] points out a problem with this view of rules, discussed below.

If we look at an arrow like this: ➡ then of itself, it means nothing. Its meaning as a symbol, which points in the direction indicated by the triangle at one end, is given to it *only* through the interpretation of the person looking at it. That interpretation depends on an understanding both of the symbolism of the shape and the context in which it is seen. A rule, similarly, only has a meaning through interpretation in a given context, by an individual who understands both the rule and the features of the situation that may make that rule relevant.

McDowell's discussion of this area is also instructive. He rejects the claim that actions, in practical situations, are capable of being codified into a set of rules.[7, pp.57–58] No matter how carefully one drew up the rules, there would always be cases where simply applying them to a situation would not be appropriate. The phrase that he uses, that 'one's mind on the matter was not susceptible of capture in a universal formula' neatly expresses the view that, in trying to decide what is the best thing to do, there simply are no *universal* rules. Recourse to rules, he suggests, is an attempt to find a safe haven in the face of this uncertainty, a way of finding 'an external standpoint outside our immersion in our familiar forms of life'.[7, p.63] As with Wittgenstein's arrow, while rules may well be of value, they will always require interpretation.

Carritt has a striking metaphor that is illuminating here. He suggests that where we have difficulties in deciding the right course of action, rules may be of great use, but 'their function is that of ballast rather than compass'.[40, p.115] In other words, they may help us keep to a course (which by implication he suggests that we, as moral agents, must decide ourselves) rather than direct us *precisely* where to go.

Wiggins also addresses the issue of following rules.[10, pp.222–28] He rejects an interpretation of Aristotle's practical reasoning based on a 'rule-case' syllogism. The examples given in support of this interpretation – to do with putting on cloaks or deciding to walk – are trivial, whereas the problems that require considerable thought, and involve hard choices, he suggests, are unlikely to be satisfactorily solved by simply invoking a rule, and subsuming the case under it.[10, p.228]

The Aristotelian approach to rules is an unashamedly contextual one. He uses the vivid metaphor of the Lesbian rule,[41, NE1137b30-32] a flexible metal instrument used to measure awkward shapes in building 'which adapts itself to the shape of the stone and is not rigid' to indicate that 'when the thing is indefinite, the rule also is indefinite'. Rules will always need to be adapted to particular circumstances.

General practice, with its blurry boundaries, does not generally lend itself to decisions based on rigidly applied rules. In making decisions, we need a flexibility of response to a situation that a rule-based normative ethical theory has great difficulty in providing.

Consequences and Utilitarianism

Decision making, according to consequentialist theories, should be based on looking clearly at the consequences of decisions. In the utilitarian variant of consequentialism, we merely need to look at what produces the most good, preferably in a measurable form, and decide accordingly. In many ways, this is deeply attractive, as it attempts to 'render tractable the bewildering problem of choice among heterogeneous alternatives'.[8, p.147]

Nussbaum's analysis of this 'science of measurement' (by which she means the measurement of alternative courses of action by a single quantitative standard of value) is useful here. First of all, one has to establish how one can measure the good. A quantitative measure, which can be applied to choice, is required. To make comparisons, this should be a single measure applicable in differing situations. Also, at the root of consequentialism is the claim that actions are important not in themselves but only in the ends or consequences that they produce. The usual consequence chosen is happiness or utility.[8, p.147]

Nussbaum points out some fundamental problems with this approach. The concept of happiness as a single quantifiable measurable entity is problematic, as pleasures are of many kinds, and cannot be easily compared. If one chooses utility, then we are faced with a similar problem of differing goods, which must, in some way be aggregated and compared. Thus, in applying utilitarianism, we face the difficulty of **incommensureability**, the problem of consequences that cannot be ordered by a single measure, and therefore cannot properly be compared one with another.[42, p.69]

By concentrating on the maximisation, but not the *distribution* of the good, there is the risk of creating or worsening unfairness or injustice. In using health economics, a utilitarian discipline, we constantly run this risk.[43, p.70] By insisting on maximising the good, the theory makes great demands of moral agents. Personal projects, loyalties to family and friends should be ignored in the pursuit of such maximisation. Williams,[44, p.574] in a penetrating critique, suggests that the principle of act utilitarianism, by focusing only on the consequences of an action, and ignoring the value of the action itself, undermines the integrity of the agent, as the decision on what to do is made on the basis of a calculation that appears to take no account of either the character or the personal projects of the agent. Personal integrity, he suggests, is a construct made intelligible only by our individually chosen actions, and if these are effectively divorced from our projects, as they appear to be in act utilitarianism, there is a central incoherence to the theory. This is a very telling objection. *In general practice, I suggest that to apply evidence-based medicine (based on populations) to individual patients without applying judgement, an intensely personal quality, to the situation, is to do precisely this.*

Therefore, to use such a theory to make decisions with patients in general practice does pose considerable problems. We may have difficulty deciding what the best consequence or outcome is for our patient, we may create or exacerbate injustice, and we may reduce ourselves to machines for calculating outcomes, and ignore the qualities of judgement that we can often usefully bring to bear on a situation, undermining our personal and (possibly our professional) integrity. Consequentialism is also rule-based, the simple rule being that decisions should be based only on consequences. The arguments on pages 11–12 therefore also apply.

Can Normative Ethical Theories Resolve Disagreement?

Besides these problems in practical situations, both deontological and consequentialist theories can be criticised from another standpoint. Wiggins[6, p.208] sets out this position:

a judgement [is] indispensably sustained by the perceptions and feelings and thoughts that are open to criticism that is based on norms that are open to criticism.

Thus judgement, 'the act of judging a content', while containing or permitting a degree of relativism, is always open to external attack and modification. Normative theories – deontological or consequentialist – which try to rule out subjectivity completely, he suggests have not succeeded in doing so. There will always be, in any ethical theory, the *possibility* of substantive disagreement. 'The familiar processes of reasoning, conversion and criticism', he proposes, are what we need.

A Caveat

However, this does not mean that we reject deontological or consequentialist ways of thinking out of hand, or suggest that they are of no relevance. They may well be of relevance and value, but the limitations of such ways of thinking in practical situations, discussed above, suggests that we should *start* our consideration of how to decide from an examination of the particular situation. We should use them, in Aristotle's words, in a manner that is 'appropriate to the occasion'.[41, NE1104a5-10] This is a central feature of the practical reasoning approach.

Aristotle, Virtue and Practical Reasoning

There are many different interpretations of Protagoras's maxim,[42, p.307–08] the epigraph to this chapter. I use it here only to emphasise the central place of the agent in decision making.

McDowell[7, p.50] suggests that to look at ethics from the standpoint of a normative ethical theory, as described above, is to look at it 'from the outside in'. In contrast, the Aristotelian approach to ethics is founded on the concept of the virtuous person. How to live, including the important business of choosing and making decisions, is understood, as McDowell says, 'from the inside out'.

Aristotle describes virtue thus:

Virtue, then, is a state of character concerned with choice, lying in a mean, i.e. the mean relative to us, this being determined by a rational principle, and by that principle by which the man of practical wisdom would describe it.[41, NE1106b36-1107a3] (my emphasis)

Thus, practical reasoning has a major role to play in the exercise of the virtues. (Practical reasoning is what the man of practical wisdom, the possessor of this virtue, does.)

The approach laid out here does not, however, depend on an account of the virtues. The aspect of virtue that is important is not a discussion of what the virtues are, nor an attempt at a normative virtue theory. Instead, it is based on the virtuous agent's 'sensitivity to a certain sort of requirement that situations impose on behaviour'.[7, p.51] Sheehan has described this as the agent's 'take' on a situation.[20, xi]

What the 'take' means is an ability to read or assess a situation correctly. It relies on what McDowell[7, p.51] calls 'a perceptual capacity' and Wiggins[10, p.231] calls 'situational appreciation'. Nussbaum describes it as 'some sort of complex responsiveness to the salient features of one's situation'.[8, p.146] It includes the use of imagination and the responses of the emotions. This responsiveness is influenced by experience, which brings with it judgement. Rules and consequences may well have a part to play in making decisions, but *whether* they have a part to play, and *what* that part is, is determined by the agent's judgement, his assessment of the context. This is the aspect of virtue that is important.

I now want to explore the nature of practical reasoning, and how it can help the agent choose what is the most appropriate way to act in a given situation.

Practical Reasoning

With what is practical reasoning concerned? Aristotle suggests that it 'is concerned with things human and things about which it is possible to deliberate'.[NE1141b10] Furthermore, excellence in deliberation is characterised by 'rightness in respect both of the end, the manner, and the time.'[NE1142b27-9]

He explores the nature of these concerns,[NE1112b9-12] when he suggests that we deliberate about situations in which it is not clear what we should do, about which there is doubt and indeterminacy. The sense of what he says is that in many circumstances, making decisions involves taking into account a great many factors, not all of which can be given a numerical value or weight.

He continues in this section[NE1112b11-13] to say that in complex and difficult issues, we need to consult with others, when we consider that we are 'not equal to deciding'.

If we consider medicine in the light of what Aristotle says, there is considerable sense here. Many situations in medicine, for example, which require a decision to be made, are intrinsically very complicated. In very few situations is it possible to predict the outcome with complete certainty, even with the aid of modern diagnostic tests that purport to give objective information about a patient. In general practice, where patients are often seen early in the course of an illness, certainty in diagnosis and prognosis is particularly elusive. Discussion with professional colleagues and referral to hospital is an obvious way of consulting with others in cases of difficulty.

In contrast, in some purely scientific areas, he suggests in NE1112b1-3, deliberation is unnecessary because the nature of the subject is exact and neither needs, nor admits of deliberation. Such things include spelling and mathematics.[NE1112b22-23]

What makes a good deliberator? Aristotle states that the:

man who is without qualification good at deliberating is the man who is capable of aiming in accordance with calculation at the best for man of things attainable in action.[NE1141b12-14]

This passage suggests that deliberation has to have an aim, and that aim is 'the best.' The *practical* aspect of practical reasoning is clearly revealed in the qualifying clause 'attainable in action'. We are not dealing here with ideas of the good derived from and resting in abstraction, but with the practical and difficult business of making decisions. This is further emphasised by the use of the verb 'to aim', which indicates that while it is important to *direct* our efforts to achieve the best, that may not be and indeed rarely is, achievable. He elaborates on this, stating that good deliberation is 'rightness with regard to the expedient'.[NE1142b26]

The matter of defining what is expedient is complex. One indication of Aristotle's view on this is laid out in NE1097b6-16, where he suggests that the complete good for man is that which achieves happiness. However, this is achieved not by oneself, 'liv(ing) a solitary life', but through recognition that man is a social animal. Hence, the best good for an individual includes one's own happiness as well as an appreciation of and the achievement of the good of others. These others may include 'parents, children, wife, and in general, friends and fellow citizens, since man is born for citizenship'.[NE1097b10-12] In discussing practical reasoning in medicine, it seems obvious that the good of our patients should be, in large measure, the aim of our deliberation. However, there may also be other important but perhaps subsidiary aims, such as the sustaining of the general practitioner through a taxing, demanding career, and the careful husbanding of moderately scarce resources. The subtlety and power of Aristotle's thinking is well illustrated by his acknowledgement of this complexity.

At NE1141b15-19, Aristotle suggests a large role for practical reasoning in human affairs by suggesting that practical reasoning is not:

concerned with universals only. It must also recognise the particulars; for it is practical, and practice is concerned with particulars.

This suggests that practical reasoning is the correct approach *both* for matters of policy and for making particular, individual decisions, also discussed by Wiggins.[10, p.225] However, Aristotle does qualify this in NE1141b23-24, when he states that in some areas to which practical reasoning applies, as in medicine, there is a 'controlling kind' that must be taken into account in decision making. In Irwin's translation of this passage,[46] he has 'ruling science' for 'controlling kind'.

The idea of a ruling science can be taken as a reminder that even though a practical reasoning approach needs to take into account particular circumstances, there may well be principles or even rules which act as a kind

---

xi   My understanding of this connection between virtue and reason, and of McDowell's account owes a great deal to discussions with Mark Sheehan.

of framework for decision-making, and which may reduce to some degree the uncertainty involved and the scope of the deliberation. As discussed on pages 11–12, all rules need contextual interpretation.

In general practice, as discussed in chapter one, it is common to use EBM in the form of an analysis of randomised controlled trials or a guideline[47] to inform a decision about a patient. However, such a 'ruling science' certainly does not dictate what should be done in every case of a medical condition referred to in the evidence. As McDowell[7, p.58] suggests, 'a mechanical application of the rules would strike one as wrong'. The evidence may be important in shaping and directing the GP's response to, and decision in, a particular situation, guided by the situational appreciation discussed above, and considered in detail below.

To summarise therefore, Aristotle's view is that we need deliberation where there is uncertainty about things of human concern, and where we are trying to achieve the best possible in a given situation, acknowledging that there is often, in the difficult business of living, no antecedently prescribed way forward.

Practical Reasoning: A Modern Account

This section presents an account of practical reasoning drawn from recent literature substantially based on Aristotle's Nicomachean Ethics. There are two related aspects of this: the priority of the particular and situational appreciation, which includes imagination and the appropriate engagement of the emotions.

The priority of the particular

I have suggested on page 12 that no normative ethical theory can rule out the possibility of disagreement in practical situations. Practical situations each and all have their own distinctive peculiarities. Normative theories simply cannot take account of all of these, and, in deliberating, we need to consider of prime importance the individual situation with all its complexities and contingencies, rather than giving priority to general rules and principles. The phrase 'the priority of the particular' above is that of Nussbaum,[8, p.155] and the following discussion is based on her work.

In discussing the idea that virtue of character is a mean, and that actions based on virtues may be praiseworthy or blameworthy depending on how far they stray from the mean, Aristotle states:

> But up to what point and to what extent a man must deviate before he becomes blameworthy it is not easy to determine by reasoning . . .; such things depend on particular facts, *and the decision rests with perception*.[NE1109b20-23] (my emphasis)

Nussbaum suggests three aspects of decision making that point to the need to concentrate on particular facts and situations, rather than on general or universal rules.[8, pp.160–62] These are: the essential indeterminacy and indefiniteness inherent in particular situations, the problem of dealing with the new and unprecedented, and the uniqueness of each particular situation. It is arguable that each of these represents a different but related facet of particularity.

Indeterminacy and indefiniteness

In a discussion on law in NE1137b13-29, Aristotle states that the law can be used to make decisions that will generally, but by no means always, be correct. This is not the fault of the law but 'in the nature of the thing, since the matter of practical affairs is of this kind from the start'.

In other words, there is in law, as in all other areas of reasoning, no 'one size fits all' basis for decisions. In making particular judgements, a good judge will require flexibility of thinking.

This passage touches on an important feature of situations: that they include indeterminate and indefinite elements that resist capturing in universal rules or formulae. While acknowledging that 'we must act according to the right rule',[NE1103b33] Aristotle qualifies this by stating that:

> the whole account of matters of conduct must be given in outline and not precisely . . . matters concerned with conduct and questions of what is good for us have no fixity, any more than matters of health.[NE1104a1-5]

Wiggins[10, p.233] further suggests that it is an intrinsic and inescapable aspect of being human to face 'an indefinite or infinite range of contingencies' with necessarily limited skills and powers to deal with them.

In considering the particular in this way, it is important to note that Aristotle is not denying that general rules may be used in decision making. However, deliberation *starts* from a consideration of the particular. Only in considering the particular situation in all its complexity does the agent have a basis for making good decisions.

Dealing with new situations

In addition to the indeterminate, indefinite nature of the practical, Nussbaum[8, pp.160-61] suggests a further reason for the priority of the particular. Life is not a steady state, but a process of continuous change. As Heraclitus said, 'People step into the same rivers, and different waters flow onto them'.[xii, 48, p.633] Decision making must take change into account. We are confronted with new situations every day, for which previous general rules or principles may well leave us unprepared.

This point is also stressed by Wiggins.[10, p.232] He suggests that life challenges us continually with new situations, which require a continuing responsiveness, not an unthinking, rigid application of previously held views, rules or principles. It is entirely appropriate that these new situations may change our ideas on what the correct course of action ought to be. It is arguable that it is only this way of reasoning that enables us to learn about and

---

xii This image can be understood either as indicating an underlying consistency and permanence (the same river), or of continuing change (different waters).[48, p.640] The fact, of course, is that in nature both are true. As a metaphor in this context, it illustrates that the agent has to be aware of both the similarities (which can help with judgement on when to use rules, and which rules to use), and the differences between situations.

respond to the world in a way that acknowledges that unremitting and continuing change are part of our existence.[xiii]

The uniqueness of the particular

It is also an important feature of particular situations that, even if there are general rules and principles that may apply to them, they are all, in some way, unique. Nussbaum[8, p.162] cites Aristotle's example of Milo the wrestler, a famous athlete, to illustrate this.[NE1106b1-5] Milo, being presumably a large, well-built, athletic person, will require more food than a small, elderly, or lazy person. Nussbaum suggests that while it is arguable that all wrestlers of Milo's size and build will require a similar diet, there will always be aspects of Milo's history and physiology that will demand an individual assessment and prescription of his diet.

Of course, this is also true in medicine. To illustrate the problem of over-simplistic application of EBM, Greenhalgh[11, p.396] suggests that just because the average woman in the UK fits a size 16 dress, it does not mean that all women should have to wear this size. (Also a woman of size 16, indeed, may *choose* to wear a size 14 or 18, dependent on *her* assessment of the situation.) Similarly, the randomised controlled trials on which EBM is based cannot take into account *all of the relevant circumstances of every patient* to whom the trial may apply. One of these circumstances is the view of the patient, who may be just as likely to have a strong view on her treatment as on her dress size. Rogers[49] in a review of ethical implications of the use of guidelines, suggests potential conflicts between their use and respect for patient autonomy. Decisions, of course, still have to be made, and it is important that a consideration of this uniqueness does not paralyse the agent's capability to make these decisions.

Situational appreciation: deliberative specification

Aristotle's view is that practical reasoning is about dealing with particular situations, which must be *perceived correctly*. Nussbaum[8, p.146] suggests this perception or **aisthesis** is 'some sort of complex responsiveness to the salient features of one's concrete situation'. Few situations consist only of easily and simply perceived elements; most have layers of nuance and complexity, which require deliberation. Wiggins[10, p.231] suggests that in exercising this capacity in a given situation, an agent will, 'prompt the imagination to play on the question and let it activate in reflection and thought experiment whatever concerns and passions it should activate'. I shall return to the issues of imagination and passions. Important here is that such a process, according to Wiggins 'requires a high order of situational appreciation'.

What this means is that, through this process, the agent provisionally identifies the relevant concerns about the situation. However, to make a decision well, these concerns have to be further specified in order to disentangle which are of importance in achieving the desired end, and which are not. Furthermore, some concerns may be more relevant than others and these must, in some way, be arranged. Wiggins describes this process as 'deliberative specification'.

In a situation where what is desired in terms of outcome is unclear, as described above, the process of deliberative specification helps to clarify what 'qualifies as an adequate and practically realisable specification of what would satisfy this want'.[10, p.225] In other words, the 'want' – what constitutes the end – becomes clear during the process of deliberative specification. During the process, the agent is considering what means can help to bring this about, but the complexities that arise during this process can lead to reconsidering, a number of times, what best or *most practically* specifies the end. The business is therefore not one of simply deciding the process of reaching end B by means A, but of deciding *both* what specifies the best outcome and what is the best way to reach it. So the process is not just about achieving the end, but also about defining what constitutes the end.

Wiggins also states that allied to this is the impossibility of developing a general or universal theory or set of rules that will deal with all these layers of nuance and complexity, characterised by indefiniteness, novelty and uniqueness as described above. This is not to suggest that the agent will not be aware of and will not take into account in his deliberation theories, rules, principles and consequences, all of which may, to a degree, be relevant (see pages 11–12).

How is this end to be achieved? Wiggins[10, p.233] suggests that it is achieved by looking at the relationship of the agent, the available universal knowledge about the situation and the relevant particular knowledge. The apotheosis of practical reasoning, he suggests, obtains when an agent identifies the greatest number of 'genuinely pertinent concerns and genuinely relevant considerations' in a particular situation, and distils out of these the essence of those that apply best. The decision or judgement is therefore made without pre-judging the situation in the light of a rule or principle which may not be relevant in the context.

Here, in applying judgement, is where the importance of experience becomes apparent. At NE1142a12-15, Aristotle states that:

> While young men become geometricians and mathematicians and wise in matters like these, it is thought that a young man of practical wisdom cannot be found. The cause is that such wisdom is concerned not only with universals but with particulars, which become familiar from experience, but a young man has no experience, for it is length of time that gives experience.

At NE1143b10-15, he suggests that:

> we ought to attend to the undemonstrated sayings and opinions of experienced and older people or people of practical wisdom not less than to

---

[xiii] This is nowhere more true than the world of medicine where new diseases and treatments arise all the time. Not only does the science of medicine change, but the development of new theoretical approaches to the subject, such as those of evidence-based and narrative-based medicine, and the development of a new GMS contract require an ongoing flexibility of response from the practitioner. This will be further discussed in chapter three.

demonstrations; for because experience has given them an eye they see aright.

Young people need time to gain experience; through the experience of seeing many different situations over a period of time, a person acquires the ability – 'an eye' – to identify relevant concerns and pertinent considerations. Aristotle also makes the interesting point that we should pay attention to the *undemonstrated* sayings and opinions of those of practical wisdom. The 'perceptual capacity' discussed earlier is enhanced by long experience of particulars; these are reflected in judgement. However, judgement cannot be simply shown by, or reduced to, demonstration.

Nussbaum[8, p.166] further reflects the importance of experience when she says 'experience is concrete and is not exhaustively summarisable in a system of rules'.

Experience and judgement are of great importance in correct decision making in general practice. Recent literature[11, pp.395–400] discusses how to combine evidence (demonstration) and 'intuition'. This will be further discussed in chapter three.

In summary therefore, a very significant aspect of the approach is the concept of situational appreciation. What this ensures is that when decisions are made, they reflect the concerns and the objectives of the agent, the salient features of the particular situation and the way in which any general or universal principles, guidelines or rules should be brought to bear on the situation.

Situational appreciation: the role of the imagination and the emotions

In the process of deliberative specification, Wiggins[10, p.231] suggests that the agent, in exercising situational appreciation, should 'prompt the imagination to play on the question'. Imagination therefore has an important part to play in connection with practical reasoning. Nussbaum[8, p.168] suggests that **phantasia,** in the way in which that term is used by Aristotle:

works closely in tandem with memory, enabling the creature to focus on absent experienced items in their concreteness, and even to form new combinations, not yet experienced, from items that have entered sense experience.

This sort of deliberative *phantasia,* she suggests, enables an agent to compare particulars, past and present, with one another, rather than with general rules or principles. This is surely very close, if not identical to the 'imagination' that Wiggins describes. Only through this process can agents use their experiences of previous situations, decisions and outcomes – good and bad – in a way that helps them to shed light on the situations before them. It also helps to explain why experience is of great importance in practical reasoning, as only through experience does the agent acquire a store of such items. Memory itself, though necessary, is insufficient, as the agent must be able not only to remember, but also to identify which remembered items are of importance, and which are not, an important aspect of deliberative specification.

Wiggins[10, p.231] states that the agent should, 'let [the imagination] activate in reflection and thought experiment whatever concerns and passions it should activate'. Why passions? While Wiggins acknowledges that passions or emotions have a place in practical reasoning, it is Nussbaum who explains why and how they are intrinsic to the process. She takes her cue from Aristotle's view that virtue is expressed both in feelings and in actions, and that having these feelings:

at the right times, with reference to the right objects, towards the right people, with the right motive and in the right way, is what is both intermediate or best, and this is characteristic of virtue.[NE1106b21-4]

Aristotle says that the virtuous person feels *appropriately*; these feelings are specific to an object or a situation, and constitute an integral part of the situational appreciation that is at the heart of practical reasoning. The *aisthesis* or situational appreciation that is central to practical reasoning therefore requires the responses not only of the intellect, but also of the emotions, which offer a sort of answering response to that of the intellect.

If one considers the process of deliberative specification outlined by Wiggins, specifying the end or outcome to be achieved requires a consideration by both the intellect and the emotions. This is also central to Nussbaum's understanding of choosing.

The place of emotions in deliberation is of particular importance in general practice, a discipline founded on relationships.[5, p.434] This will be further considered in chapter three. Blackburn[50, pp.125–33] in his detailed account of practical reasoning, rejects the idea that emotions are disruptive influences in thinking, and suggests instead that our attachment to 'long-term goals' is a state partially determined by our emotions, 'fear of failure, anger at obstacles' for example. This seems to fit with the Aristotelian position that 'choice is either desiderative reason or ratiocinative desire'.[NE1139b3-5]

Blackburn also discusses empirical evidence from individuals with traumatic brain damage causing a dissociation of affect from cognition, (including the well-known case of Phineas Gage) to support the view that such a dissociation leads to a complete inability to make decisions that make external sense. Without emotional engagement, no alternative, in such an individual, makes any more sense than any other, and behaviour becomes bizarre and incomprehensible.

Normative ethical theories and emotions

It is a distinctive feature of Aristotle's thinking on ethics that it includes such a significant place for emotions and feelings. By comparison, deontological thinking, which concerns itself mainly with obligations, may be well suited to legal contracts and political theories, but seems to ignore the importance of emotions and feelings, although those are generally considered to be part of a well-lived life. Beauchamp and Childress[11, pp.354–55] suggest that it 'overemphasises law, underemphasises relationships'. Such thinking seems to reduce all relationships to relationships between strangers, rather than between professionals, friends or family members.

Utilitarianism also has little place for emotions or feelings. If we are to base our actions solely on what maximises happiness, then we may be forced to ignore close personal ties based on relationships and feelings. Giving all our surplus money to charities in developing countries when our own parents may be needy (but not as needy as those in Africa) is a simple example. This seems to ignore or undermine the personal projects and commitments that are central to our lives. Williams,[44, p.575] in discussing an example of the well-known 'horrific act' objection to utilitarianism, points out that part of the horror of such acts involves agents ignoring feelings such as revulsion, which are not given weight in a utilitarian calculus.

Practical Reasoning: Summary and Objections

To summarise, therefore, I have suggested that we need practical reasoning in situations where the outcome is unclear and uncertain, and where we are trying to achieve the best outcome possible under the circumstances. Practical reasoning requires that the agent gives priority to the particular features of the situation before him or her, and applies a well-developed perceptual capacity or situational appreciation – derived from experience and training – to it. An important part of this capacity is the appropriate use of imagination and finely tuned emotions.

Objections to situational appreciation

The main objection to this account is put succinctly by Wiggins:[10, p.237]

> *Everything that is hard has been permitted to take refuge in the notion of aisthesis, or situational appreciation ... And in aisthesis, as Aristotle says, explanations give out.*

The strength of the notion of situational appreciation is that it expresses the depth and complexity of agents' interactions with the world around them. In an earlier paper, Wiggins[45, p.96] suggests that *aisthesis* represents a 'no man's land' between initial assessment of what is ('unweighted initial appreciation') and a completed 'practical decision'. This must represent, as Aristotle states[NE1139b3-5] and Wiggins explains,[10, p.237] the desires and aims of the agent as well as a consideration of external notions of what may constitute a good outcome. It may also include the sensible assessment of rules and principles.

Unlike utilitarian reasoning, which is subject to the strictures described by Williams[44, p.574] and discussed on page 12, situational appreciation allows the essential connection between the 'agent's desires and perceptions of how things are in the world about him, his subjective motivation and the objective limitations of his situation'.[28, p.178] Thus, the approach does not ignore either duties or obligations, or maximising the good, but acknowledges that these ways of looking at the world represent important, but not necessarily dominant features in the landscape of making decisions.

To use another metaphor, it does not depend on Procrustean[xiv] theories that attempt to mould either the agent or the world into a bed which fits neither of them well. Instead, the approach offers what Aristotle[NE1104a5-10] describes as 'what is appropriate to the occasion'.

The issue of indeterminacy and indefiniteness

The Aristotelian view that practical situations will always contain indeterminate and indefinite elements is also open to criticism. I use indeterminate here in the sense of having no certain or fixed value, and indefinite as being without clearly marked outlines or limits.[51]

That may have been the case in 360BC, it can be said, but in the twenty-first century, we have a welter of objective data and information from the biological, psychological, social and economic sciences that can be used to provide data and knowledge about many situations. This means that often, indeterminacy can be minimised, and indefiniteness at least reduced in scope. This makes choosing easier, and means that we should not now have to take refuge in such antediluvian vagueness.

There are several responses to this. Data may, of course, be inaccurate. Also, it may not be truly objective, but may have been selectively obtained for specific circumstances, and to fulfil certain demands. Much scientific data is derived from studies of populations. It is commonplace in the biological and social sciences to apply data from one population to another, when there may be subtle but substantial differences between those populations.

To intrapolate from population data to decisions for individuals may be to indulge in the ecological fallacy. This is to falsely assume that conclusions derived from the population data will apply to each individual in that dataset.[xv]

Such hard quantitative data, no matter how accurate, can only describe certain selected elements of a situation. This is the basis of **reductionist** science.[34, pp.2-5] While such science has achieved a huge amount for humankind over the past two centuries, it is important to be aware that it has done so by selecting out certain elements of a situation to study.

Scientific data is fact. In the context of general practice consultations, it is very important not to ignore hard data, in the form of evidence and guidelines, which will give the GP important information about how to manage Mrs Smith's arthritis, diabetes, high blood pressure or breast cancer, for example (see Appendix one). However, when we make a decision about what we *ought* to do, we are also deciding how we assess, consider

---

xiv Procrustes, in Greek legend, was a robber of Attica, who put all his victims into an iron bed. If they were longer than the bed, he cut off the overhanging parts, and if they were shorter, he stretched them to fit.

xv Greenhalgh[33, pp.251-52] discusses this problem in detail. She quotes AN Whitehead's famous remark from 1925, when he describes this use of data as 'the fallacy of misplaced concreteness'. Stephen Jay Gould[52, p.31] reminds us that 'variation is the hard reality ... means and medians are the abstractions'. Leder[53, p.21] talks of the 'ideal of perfect presence – the immediate gaze, the unambiguous number'. The problem is essentially one of the **reification** of numbers.

or value this data. Is it objective? Is it accurate? Is it valid for this situation, for Mrs Margaret Smith today? What other data, less easy to measure but salient to this situation must I take into account? This might include contextual information from the patient's facial expressions and body language, the verbal and non-verbal cues that are enormously important in communication in general practice. This aspect of the consultation is explored in more depth in chapter three. The claim of this chapter is that it is only through practical reasoning, which involves serious deliberation and reflection on all aspects of the individual situation, that intelligence and knowledge, derived *in part* from hard data and information, are used to make the best decisions.

Conclusion

I have outlined an approach to making decisions based on a modern conception of practical reasoning, founded on Aristotle's ethics. It is based on a focus on the particular. The central core of the approach is situational appreciation, a capacity for deliberation and reasoning on every relevant aspect of a situation. It may encompass rules and measures of outcome where these are applicable. It gives an important place to imagination and the emotions, but does not privilege them. My claim is that it represents the most comprehensive way of understanding the exciting, difficult and complex nature of our relationships with one another and with the world. It is in this world, with all its 'forms of life'[39, p.192e] that we make our decisions.

Chapter Three
Aristotle's Answer (2)
Decision Making in General Practice: The Practice of Perception

...the account of particular cases is yet more lacking in exactness; for they do not fall under any art or precept, but the agents themselves must in each case consider what is appropriate to the occasion, as happens also in the art of medicine or of navigation. Aristotle[NE1104a5-10] (my emphasis)

Can one learn this knowledge? Yes; some can. Not, however, by taking a course in it, but through experience. From time to time he gives him the right tip. This is what learning and teaching are like here. What one acquires here is not a technique; one learns correct judgements. There are also rules, but they do not form a system, and only experienced people can apply them right. Unlike calculating rules. What is most difficult here is to put this indefiniteness, correctly and unfalsified, into words.

Wittgenstein, L[39, p.193e]

Introduction

This chapter will discuss the practical reasoning approach set out in chapter two in the context of decision making in general practice. I describe this as the *practice of perception*. Practice here is not used in a technical sense, but in the everyday sense of the regular performance of a difficult task, through which skills are gradually acquired. Perception refers essentially to the situational appreciation discussed in chapter two. This is illustrated by an example (see Appendix one). First of all, however, I wish to discuss some contemporary literature on practical reasoning and clinical practice.

Narrative, Hermeneutics and Practical Reasoning

Greenhalgh's acknowledgement of the central place of interpretation in clinical practice[33, p.256] discussed in chapter one page 9, leads naturally to a consideration of hermeneutics, the detailed study of interpretation of narrative. Leder's discussion of the hermeneutics of medicine[53] is based on the doctor interpreting the 'text' of the ill person, which he divides into experiential (the illness as experienced by the patient), narrative (the patient's history), physical (the findings on examination), and instrumental (comprising the results of investigations). This deconstruction then requires the interpretive skills of the experienced doctor to make into a coherent whole in order to make the best decision. He admits that to designate medicine as hermeneutical can be considered trivial, but argues that the textual analysis elaborated in his discussion provides a way of seeing that offers clarity and insight.

The usefulness of Leder's approach is that it moves away from the biomedical model described in chapter one, and acknowledges the elements of subjectivity involved in interpretation. However, it is arguably difficult to view the patient as a series of related 'texts', and unclear whether they are intended to be merely descriptive of the clinical encounter or whether they offer a sort of prescriptive specification for decision making in medicine.

Hunter[54] suggests that the narrative of cases is the starting point from which doctors apply and modify the evidence base of medicine. All narratives need interpretation, as they are drawn from particular standpoints, and express an 'unabashedly situated subjectivity'.[54, p.306] Doctors acquire over time – through their clinical work, discussion with colleagues and reading – experience of many narratives, many clinical situations. To make clinical decisions from these narratives, Hunter suggests, we need Aristotelian ***phronesis***, defined as: 'a means of operating in the world, a matter of understanding how best to act in particular circumstances that are not (and cannot be) thoroughly expressed in general rules'.[54, p.304]

This is clearly very similar to the view of MacIntyre, who characterises the possessor of practical reasoning as 'someone who knows how to exercise judgement in particular cases'.[30, p.154]

If we now consider what Schon[55, pp.49–50] calls 'reflection-in-action' among professionals (not only doctors), he states:

Every competent practitioner can recognise phenomena – families of symptoms associated with a particular disease, peculiarities of a certain kind of building site, irregularities of materials or structures – for which he cannot give a reasonably accurate or complete description. In his day-to-day practice he makes innumerable judgements of quality for which he cannot state adequate criteria, and he displays skills for which he cannot state the rules and procedures. Even when he makes conscious use of research based theories and techniques, he is dependent on tacit recognition, judgements and skilful performances.

These definitions have many points in common. In dealing with the individual situation – Schon's 'particular disease ... certain sort of building site, irregularities of materials or structures', we are in a territory where, as discussed in chapter two (pages 11–12), rules, although they may well be of considerable relevance, cannot be simply *applied* to each and every situation. Schon's description especially has a kind of face validity for general practice, in that it describes well the uneliminable uncertainty which GPs face in their professional lives, *and the way in which they address it*.

It is the claim of this chapter that *the practice of perception* offers us an approach that adequately acknowledges both the subjectivity of interpretation and the objectivity of hard data. It is through this that the GP is able to learn how to interpret complex clinical situations, as the epigraphs to this chapter suggests. It is enabled by the doctor's experience of many similar situations over a long period of time, his understanding of the individual circumstances of that patient, *and* his understanding of the evidence base of medicine.[31] Through the exercise of the practice of perception, the GP establishes what *ought* to be done.

The Practice of Perception

I will now relate my discussion of practical reasoning in chapter two to the issue of decision making in general practice. The practice of perception rests on the priority of the particular and situational appreciation. It is founded on McWhinney's understanding of general practice, set out in chapter one. Central to this are the following: that the discipline is based on the relationship between the doctor and the patient, on individuals rather than diseases, and that it rejects both a mechanistic view of the body and the mind–body duality.

A grasp of the priority of the particular

> *The closer we are to a person, the more we are aware of their individual particulars, and the more difficult it is to think of them as members of a class.*
>
> McWhinney[5, p.433]

> *Narrative knowledge in scientific medicine owes its tenacity to the profession's duty to make sense of the presentation of illness by a particular patient.*
>
> Hunter[54, p.310]

These quotations illustrate the need for the focus, in the clinical encounter, to be on the particular case, the individual patient. In chapter two, I discussed three aspects of the priority of the particular: indeterminacy and indefiniteness, dealing with new situations, and the uniqueness of the particular. How are these relevant in consultations between GPs and patients?

Indeterminacy

Most clinical situations contain indeterminate, hard to define elements. The patient's experience and the clinical history cannot be simply defined and measured. The experience of the patient is expressed in words and gestures that express, implicitly or explicitly, his or her *interpretation* of symptoms or events. The patient's story expresses his or her experience within the context of an illness *yet to be defined*, and requires further interpretation by the doctor and the patient together.

The physical findings and the test results tend to fall within the general description of evidence-based medicine, and are generally quantifiable and determinate. However, as discussed on pages 17–18, these will also always require interpretation for the individual circumstances.

Dealing with the new

Only by looking carefully at the particular can we recognise new clinical situations, which happen regularly. If we look at a patient and see, among the diagnostic possibilities, only conditions that we have seen before, we risk missing the new disease or the unusual, unexpected presentation. The appearance of many completely new diseases over the past twenty years (HIV, *E. coli* O157, new variant Creutzfeldt-Jakob disease, severe acute respiratory syndrome) illustrates this very well. We need a flexibility of response, based on keen observation of what is before us, not pre-interpreted through a rigid framework of thinking only about what *has been*. We also need the same flexibility to continually refresh our ideas about medicine, the lens through which we see the clinical world. The continually developing and changing ideas discussed in chapter one – Balint, evidence-based medicine, McWhinney's analysis – mean that, as we go through a professional life, not only does our gaze have to reflect changing diseases, but also changing conceptions of who we are and what we, as doctors, do. This flexibility, which includes a capacity for improvisation, is important in both responding to *and* developing new ideas.

Uniqueness

Each clinical encounter is unique. In chapter two, I suggested that practical reasoning necessarily starts with the consideration of a particular situation, and discussed the relevance of this to the clinical encounter.

The two quotations at the start of this section illustrate the importance of the GP having a particular person or patient as their focus. The patient's *experience* of an illness, discussed above, is unique to that individual, that encounter. In general practice, as McWhinney[5] suggests, the engagement of the GP is based on a *relationship with an individual patient, not a disease*. The 'situation' that situational appreciation considers in general practice, will therefore include seeing the person, the particular patient, before the clinical content of the case is established. The situation is therefore not purely a clinical one, and the GP will be aware of many family and social issues that impact on and affect the patient's encounter with the GP (see Dr Lawrence's problem, Appendix one). The clinical encounter therefore cannot be objectified, the gaze should be both wide and deep, and the case will always have features that are dissimilar to other clinical encounters. The sense that McWhinney seems to express is that the GP should be, in a phrase of Henry James, 'a person on whom nothing is lost'.[8, p.177]

Situational Appreciation

The feature that makes a general practitioner unique (even in the medical domain) is the ability to sort the unsorted – differentiate the undifferentiated problem within the domain of life, the universe and everything.

Purves [9, p.39]

This section deals with the core of decision making in general practice, the central problem of which is well expressed by Purves above. GPs deal with a huge range of conditions: the management of ingrowing toenails, the assessment of suicide risk in a depressed patient, the immediate care of meningococcal meningitis are examples of the extremes. Furthermore, our decisions have to reflect not just the immediate, but also the long-term interests of that patient.

Evidence and intuition: the place of deliberative specification

How is this 'sorting' to be done? In the course of a clinical encounter, we acquire a large amount of undifferentiated information – the patient's experience expressed as a story, physical findings, and laboratory results – all of which require interpretation.

To start with, some of the information may be construed as evidence. This may include physical findings and measurements of a patient's cholesterol, blood pressure, glucose, blood counts or other parameters that may be understood through measurement. These measurements may well be of considerable significance in decision making. This empirical *evidence* may well help to *specify* what will achieve the best outcome for that patient. When Sackett[31] talks of 'the conscientious, explicit, and judicious use of current best evidence in making decisions about the care of individual patients', he is saying strongly that when evidence is available, its consideration should constitute an important part of the process of deliberative specification for that situation, with that patient.

However, the interpretation of the *patient's story*, being concerned with the particular case, must also play a part in deliberative specification, and in many cases, it may play a more central part than the evidence. The relative weight attached to these elements in deliberative specification is a matter of judgement in each particular situation.[xvi]

The process of deliberative specification not only clarifies what is going on during the clinical encounter, but also establishes what the appropriate course of action in that situation is and what the outcome should be. It is therefore at the very core of situational appreciation.

Greenhalgh's discussion of intuition in general practice[12] is relevant here. She suggests that it[xvii] has the following features:

· rapid, unconscious process
· context sensitive
· comes with practice
· involves selective attention to small details
· cannot be reduced to cause and effect logic (i.e. B happened because of A)
· addresses, integrates and makes sense of multiple complex pieces of data.

Greenhalgh points out that intuition and evidence-based medicine are not in conflict, but are complementary. Intuition is necessary to interpret and contextualise evidence.

The close parallels between intuition and situational appreciation are evident. The focus on the particular context, the importance of experience in focusing the attention of the agent on detail, avoiding excessive reliance on rules and algorithms and the acknowledgement of complexity[xviii] are present in both. Furthermore, empirical studies of ways in which professionals of different levels of experience work[56, pp.16–51] clearly show that while novice practitioners adhere rigidly to rules and have little 'situational perception',[12] experienced practitioners who use intuition no longer follow rules or guidelines rigidly. Instead, they rely on judgements that they themselves can rarely explain clearly and rationally. This, of course, reflects Wiggins'[10] analysis of *aisthesis* or situational appreciation, when, he indicates, 'explanations give out'. This is the 'black box' aspect of intuition or situational appreciation. There is here an uneliminable measure of subjectivity, defensible primarily because there is, in these clinical situations, simply no other way forward. In considering many such situations, the fact is that we often understand much more than we can explain, either to others or ourselves. Such tacit knowledge[5] is of great importance in general practice.

Aristotle's views on experience[NE1142a12-15, NE1143b10-15] are discussed in chapter two and are clearly of great relevance here. In particular, his view that we should listen to the 'undemonstrated sayings and opinions' of those of experience, is given weight by these empirical studies. Experience contributes to judgement by giving those who have seen many different situations 'an eye' for seeing what should be done and guides the process of deliberative specification.

Experience brings with it long exposure to many particular situations. Thus:

Practical wisdom ... must also recognise the particulars; for it is practical, and practice is concerned with particulars. This is why some who

---

xvi Normal electrocardiographs and cholesterol levels, for example, cannot exclude a diagnosis of coronary heart disease, which is often made solely on the history given by the patient.
xvii The late Dr Janet Heyes has suggested that intuition is 'the ability to see round corners'.
xviii There is a growing literature on complex adaptive systems and medicine.[1,2,3] Wilson *et al*,[3] in a discussion on complexity and clinical care, give examples of how tools or techniques – provocative questioning, experiment, intuition – can be used to help make decisions in clinical encounters. However, a decision on which technique to use in a particular situation obviously cannot be made on standard scientific criteria, and it is hard to escape the conclusion that the whole process has to be underwritten by something like a practical reasoning approach if it is to make sense. Complexity theory in general practice, therefore, may in fact reflect a heavily disguised Aristotelian approach.

do not know, and especially those who have experience, are more practical than those who know.[NE1141b15-20]

Aristotle is saying here that knowledge of particulars is often more important, *in practice*, than theoretical knowledge, a point also made by W. James,[5, p.434] who suggests that 'a large acquaintance with particulars often makes us wiser than the possession of abstract formulas, however deep'.

Situational appreciation: the role of the imagination and the emotions

the doctor's attention should be outward towards the patient, and his feeling with, or his compassion for, the patient should be in an imaginative grasp of the patient's whole situation.

Downie[57, p.72]

Imagination

In chapter two, I discussed the role of the imagination and emotions in practical reasoning. In clinical situations, to grasp the 'whole situation' of the patient, Downie suggests, we need imagination.

The Aristotelian capacity for 'deliberative phantasia'[8, p.169] a sort of imagining, seems to enable the GP to do this. It is a capacity that enables the doctor to look at what is happening during an encounter in the light of previous similar consultations with this and other patients. It also includes the capacity to imagine what patients are themselves experiencing. Nussbaum describes this as 'the ability to link several imaginings or perceptions together'. It is not merely memory, as it involves a degree of discrimination, enabling the selection of which remembered items are of importance, and of how much importance.

It also enables us to imagine the possible future outcomes of differing courses of action, based on our past experience of what has gone well and what has gone badly. In Nussbaum's view,[xix] the Aristotelian conception of imagining is necessarily concrete, and therefore lends itself particularly to the understanding of complex, many-faceted, ill-defined situations, such as those that occur every day in general practice.

Thus, imagination enables the comparison of particular to particular. This is very different to an approach based on the assessment of the *evidence* alone, which always compares the particular to the general. Wiggins describes situational appreciation, discussed above, as requiring the 'prompt' of imagination[10, p.231] to 'activate' the process of deliberative specification described above.

This imaginative grasp can give GPs important information about patients' predicaments, both by enabling them to understand how similar illnesses have affected others in the past, by enabling them to understand what patients are going through, and by helping them to predict how the course of patients' illnesses may affect those patients. It relies on experience, but is also important in the *accumulation* of experience and the expression of judgement.

Imagination, however, is not, by itself, enough. Downie also suggests that part of the imaginative grasp should be 'feeling with, and compassion for the patient'.

Emotions

Greenhalgh and Hurwitz[32, p.11] suggest pessimistically that 'modern medicine lacks a metric for existential qualities like inner hurt, despair, hope, grief and moral pain which frequently accompany and indeed often constitute the illnesses from which people suffer.' 'Metric', a quantitative term, may not be the most appropriate here.[xx]

I think that the problem described by Greenhalgh and Hurwitz may stem from a lack of emotional engagement with the patient by the GP. This can be demonstrated by considering what happens when emotional engagement is absent. It is illustrated by the problem of 'burn out' among GPs, and the consequences for their patients, well described by Macnaughton.[57, p.72]

When a GP becomes 'burnt out', he deals with his patients in a way that leads to their depersonalisation. This means that the patient is treated not as an individual with an illness and with worries and concerns about how that illness may affect her or him, but merely as an example of a disease state. The GP reverts to a simple biomedical model (see chapter one). This usually happens because, after long exposure to the needs of individuals, the GP feels the need to protect him- or herself from the emotional consequences of the patient's distress.

This phenomenon, further explored by Kirwan and Armstrong[58] can therefore be said to be due to an apparent *deficiency* of feeling by the GP for the patient's predicament. It can only be avoided by awareness by doctors of their own emotions during their work, and continual seeking an appropriate level of emotional engagement with the patient, often over a long time.

However, an excess of emotional response can interfere with a proper understanding of a clinical encounter as much as a deficiency. Aristotle's view on feelings,[NE1106b21-24] discussed in chapter two, is paraphrased by Nussbaum[8, p.169] as 'feel(ing) the appropriate emotions about what he or she chooses'. In other words, the right amount of emotional response, neither too little nor too much. McWhinney describes this as 'detached involvement'.[60] (It is illustrated in Dr Lawrence's problem in Appendix one.)

I believe that this shows the need to include emotional awareness in practical reasoning, as something complementary to intellectual appreciation. Neither is privileged; both are necessary. Balint first explored this area in general practice.[17, chs. XIV–XV] McWhinney[5] makes

---

xix Greenhalgh[12, p.398] summarises some empirical evidence that supports Nussbaum's view. This evidence suggests that the way that memory stores clinical content is in the form of narrative rather than 'structured collections of abstracted facts.'

xx Poetry offers a better way of expressing and encompassing the problems referred to by Greenhalgh and Hurwitz. Attila Jozsef's poem,[59] *It hurts a lot:*
  Healthy people,
  Fall and crumble,
  Mumble to her: it hurts a lot.
  Metricity has no place here.

the point that experience, which is of great importance in making judgements, 'engages our feelings as well as our intellect.' He is reflecting Blackburn's view[50, pp.125-33] that cognition often makes no sense without emotional engagement.

The emotions enable GPs to know how to focus their work. Nussbaum describes the emotions as 'modes of vision, or recognition', as an important part of *knowing* a situation. Thus, they are not primitive forces, but should be used by GPs to guide their responses to a particular situation to achieve the best outcome for the patient.[8, p.170]

Emotion and loss

Medicine is, at the very deepest level, concerned with loss, or the possibility of loss. In many illnesses and consultations, GPs deal with patients who are afraid of loss: loss of function due to illness or ageing, loss associated with the stigma of a disease, loss of employment, friends or family, or even their own lives. It is also important to be aware that a consultation that seems to be about a minor symptom may have been interpreted by the patient as an indicator of serious, perhaps fatal disease – heart disease or cancer. The role of the GP is more often to exclude serious illness than to diagnose it. That role, however, is a hugely important one for the patient.

At the very heart of meaning in life, is this knowledge of the possibility, and in the end, the inevitability of loss. Loss will affect our attachment to the long-term goals of our lives, which Blackburn[50, p.129] argues, is a state partly determined by our emotions. There are, therefore, inevitably emotional elements to loss that must be acknowledged and dealt with in a way appropriate to the situation.

Relational empathy, imagination and emotional engagement

It is heartening to see that recent empirical work by Mercer *et al.* has started to show the importance of imagination and emotional engagement to quality of care. They[64] suggest that empathy is 'a complex, multi-dimensional concept that has moral, cognitive, motive and behavioural components'. These – Morse's components of empathy[65] – are summarised below.

Table 3.1 Morse's components of empathy

Component	Definition
Emotive	The ability to subjectively experience and share in another's psychological state or intrinsic feelings
Moral	An internal altruistic force that motivates the practice of empathy
Cognitive	The helper's intellectual ability to identify and understand another person's feelings and perspectives from an objective stance
Behavioural	Communicative response to convey understanding of another's perspective

In a further paper, Mercer *et al.*[66] suggest that the importance of each of these components to the clinical encounter is not well understood. The discussion below offers a brief exploration of how they may connect.

In the context of the discussion on pages 22–23, moral empathy can be regarded as a key element of the motivating force behind the GP's desire to help his or her patient. What Morse describes as cognitive empathy would seem to be very similar to the use of imagination and to Nussbaum's[8] understanding of Aristotle's *deliberative phantasia*, explored on page 16, and page 22 in a GP context. The 'identification and understanding of another's feelings' (see Morse's definition above) is essentially what she describes as 'the capacity to imagine what the patient herself is experiencing'. The notion of true objectivity, however, is highly questionable in this context, as one doctor's cognitive empathy may not be another's, and only the patient truly understands his or her feelings and perspectives. It is therefore arguably difficult to separate cognitive from emotive empathy, but easy to see that both elements, whether they are truly separable or not, contribute to an appropriate engagement with the patient, and are necessary for an in-depth understanding of that patient's situation. Behavioural empathy should be conveyed in the course of the consultation with the patient, and is a practical demonstration of emotional engagement or involvement.

Principles and Situational Appreciation

It is a distinctive feature of the practice of perception that, as discussed previously, it looks at how to act from 'the inside out'.[7, p.51] It relies on the capacity of the GP to read a situation well, and act accordingly.

In contrast, the standard approach in medical ethics, advocated by Beauchamp and Childress,[11, chs. 1, 3-6] is based on the four principles of medical ethics: respect for autonomy, beneficence, **non-maleficence** and justice – ethics from the outside in.

However, it would be a mistake to consider that these principles are given no place in situational appreciation. They are considered by the experienced GP, as part of the process of deliberative specification, *as and when the situation demands*, rather than as principles to be considered in abstract, general terms, and applied to the situation. A difficulty with the four principles approach advocated by Beauchamp and Childress is deciding what to do when these principles conflict in a particular situation, as they often do. Like moral rules, the four principles cannot tell us what to do in every situation. My claim is that judging a situation correctly, under these circumstances, relies on perceptual capacity, the GP's ability to assess all relevant aspects of the situation, including, where appropriate, ethical principles. (See Appendix one, Dr Lawrence's problem.)

Achieving the best outcome

All our clinical judgements must of course *aim*,[NE1141b12-14] towards the goal of achieving the best that is achievable for *the patient before us in that situation*. 'Good action is an end, and desire aims at this' states Aristotle.[NE1139b3-6] Situational appreciation allows the essential connections between, 'the agent's desires and perceptions of how things are in the world about him, his subjective motivation and the objective limitations of his situation.[28, p.178]

In the context of general practice, our *aim or desire* will be, of course, to achieve the best that we can for the patient. However, key to how we approach this are our *perceptions, intellectual and emotional or empathetic* of the case before us, which will include the patient's story, the clinical evidence and any important principles. *Subjective motivation* refers to the GP's inclination and will to pursue that aim or desire, while *objective limitations* may include available time and resources at our disposal to address the problem. Therefore, while a desire to achieve the best for the patient is the aim of the consultation,[xxi] the outcome will always be determined by the detailed practicalities of the situation, both subjective and objective.

Perceptual Capacity and Training for General Practice

> ... a conception of right conduct is grasped, as it were, from the inside out.
> McDowell, J.[7, p.50]

How does this approach apply to training for general practice today? To enter general practice, registrars have to pass summative assessment, which comprises an MCQ, submission of an audit or project, a satisfactory trainer's report, and a video assessment.[61] Many of those entering general practice today now also take the MRCGP examination.

The criteria for video assessment as a part of summative assessment are included in Appendix two. This process is designed to ensure that future GPs have a minimum standard of competence in consulting, and this is reflected in the straightforward categories of listening, action and understanding. However, to elicit the reason(s) for attending, take appropriate action, refer when necessary, and demonstrate an understanding of the process in a logbook certainly cannot be done without possessing some capacity for perception or situational appreciation.

The scope of the MRCGP examination is very wide, and passing it requires a considerable range of skills and knowledge, higher than those needed for summative assessment. I wish to focus on one component of the examination, the assessment of a video of the GP registrar's consultations, which aims to 'assess the candidate's ability in consulting and communication skills'.[62]

The performance criteria (PC), for the assessment of the video, on which a marking schedule is based, are set out in Appendix three.

The particular, perceptual capacity and the MRCGP video assessment

It is self-evident that a GP consultation requires a grasp of *the priority of the particular* as defined and discussed on page 20. It is only through this that we can, as Hunter[54, p.310] suggests, understand what the patient is saying, through a focus on that patient on that day, in that place. This focus means not viewing the patient as a 'case' of angina, or diabetes or, worse, a 'social problem', for that is to give priority to the *general*, a single aspect of that patient's medical or social history, which may or may not be important for this consultation.

If we go through the performance criteria individually, we can see how important perceptual capacity is. In eliciting an account of the patient's symptoms (PCs 1 and 2), 'encouraging the patient's contribution' and 'responding to cues' such as distress, happiness, or a flat affect, we require an awareness of facial expression and body language *and*, equally important, an understanding of how to use this information to bring out the patient's story. This requires the careful ordering of concerns and information about the situation described by Wiggins[10] as deliberative specification, the central component of situational appreciation. It is not merely observation but is a process, requiring, as the video workbook suggests, 'active listening' and an appropriate degree of responsiveness. Similarly, exploring the patient's health understanding (PC 4) requires a subtle exploration of the patient's beliefs, dependent on perception. The middle-aged executive with mild hypertension may have a disproportionate fear of stroke; the young woman with pain in one breast may think that she has cancer; a mother may be disguising a desperate worry that her toddler with a fever and a viral rash has meningitis. To be aware of issues like these requires a degree of imagination or *deliberative phantasia*, as discussed on page 22; to respond well requires empathy or emotional engagement, to the extent that the situation demands.

Making a working diagnosis (PC 7) can only be appropriately done if the doctor has sensitively gathered sufficient information through the previous criteria. The next section, explaining the problem with the patient (PCs 8, 9, 10), requires a synthesis of the doctor's understanding and the patient's health beliefs, and a confirmation of the patient's understanding of the doctor's explanation. This requires a subtle understanding of what is 'appropriate to the occasion',[NE1104a5-10] and both imagination or *phantasia*, reflecting the doctor's understanding of what the patient may be experiencing and thinking, and on most if not all occasions, a degree of emotional engagement with the patient. Underlying all of these processes is deliberative specification.

PC 12, involving the patient in the management plan, and *how* this should be done, similarly needs knowledge of what is appropriate for that patient in particular. We know that some patients want much more involvement than others, and an assessment or what is needed for each consultation, requires considerable discernment. In concrete particulars, as Aristotle says, discernment rests on perception.[NE1109b23, 8, p.158] We perceive or become aware of many things, but we need discernment, a sort of sifting or deliberative specification of what is important for *this* case, to decide what to do with or for this particular patient.

In this chapter so far, I have argued that perceptual capacity, involving a grasp of the priority of the

---

[xxi] Those observing or criticising our work therefore should not be too concerned if our management of patients may appear inconsistent with the *evidence*, so long as it is consistent with the good of *the particular patient in that situation*.

particular, and a perceptual capacity in which imagination and emotional engagement play a substantial part, is at the core of decision making within the consultation. It is not surprising, but perhaps rather reassuring, to find that it also underpins the video assessment of the consultation in the MRCGP examination. However, whether perceptual capacity can be reduced to a checklist of points to be measured in a few consultations selected for an examination is much more debatable.

The epigraph from McDowell at the head of this section is discussed in general terms on page 12. In this crucial area of general practice, it suggests that knowing what to do and how to behave cannot just be *externally* prescribed. A holistic approach means not just the whole patient, but to an interesting degree, the whole doctor. McWhinney[5] suggests that 'we can only attend to a patient's feelings and emotions if we know our own'. Neighbour's book *The Inner Consultation*,[63] an analysis of what happens in GP–patient encounters, uses different language to explain the complexity of this process. However, the process of 'connecting' and 'rapport-building skills' that he describes are certainly characterised by the exercise of both imagination and emotional engagement with the patient.

The New General Medical Services (nGMS) Contract

That practical wisdom is not scientific knowledge is evident.[NE1142a24]

The nGMS contract,[69] which came into effect in April 2004, represents the greatest change in the way GPs are financially rewarded for their work since the inception of the NHS in 1948. There was a consensus that the previous contract, a glorious mishmash of accretions accumulated between 1948 and 2003, had run its course, and was no longer fit for purpose.

Under nGMS, all practices will be required to provide 'essential services', which are defined as:

- the management of patients who are ill or who perceive themselves to be ill, including health promotion advice as appropriate, reflecting patient choice wherever practicable
- general management of patients who are terminally ill
- management of chronic disease in the manner determined by the practice, in discussion with the patient.

GPs are now no longer responsible for care of patients outside of working hours, defined as 0800–1830h. A further major change is that all patients will now register with a practice rather than an individual doctor. In addition, 30–50% of practice income is allocated as quality payments within a Quality and Outcomes Framework (QOF). The elements of the QOF are:

- a points based system of payments for achieving targets in ten chronic disease areas
- an organisational domain covering records, communication, education and management
- additional services (cervical screening, child health surveillance and maternity and contraceptive services)
- a patient experience domain, which requires an annual survey of patients of the practice and information on consultation length.

Ethical issues

The nGMS contract is a child of the information age; the extensive data collection required is only possible using the tools of information management and technology. The collection of data represents a sort of annual rolling programme of clinical and organisational audit for the practice. Through it, NHS management controls the processes and outcomes of medical care in practices, with the aim of achieving value for money and quality of care. As Power[23] suggests, the choice of criteria for audit effectively controls what happens in medical care, especially when performance is directly linked to payment, and we need to ask whether the criteria and standards defining the new contract are appropriate.

If we look in detail at the QOF, we see that for the first time, remuneration in general practice is geared towards the achievement of targets for specific chronic diseases. These are soundly based on empirical evidence whenever such evidence exists,[67, 70] and there seems little doubt that improved management of these conditions, which include the commonest chronic medical conditions in the UK such as CHD, hypertension, diabetes and asthma, *should* improve outcomes for individuals and populations. Similarly, drivers to improve organisation within general practice are likely to contribute to an environment in which good general practice can flourish. However, the 'additional' services are for many practices, part of their day-to-day work, and it seems unlikely that their inclusion in the QOF will have a major impact on performance. Patient surveys may provide useful feedback to help improve services, although there is, as yet, only limited evidence that they do so.

Rewarding practices with booked appointments of ten minutes seems sensible, as longer consultation length is strongly associated with both enablement of patients and the patient knowing the doctor well, a proxy for continuity.[71] However, here are also wider questions about the philosophical basis of this new direction. Perhaps like any such contract, it attempts to achieve as much good as possible for a very wide range of patients in very different practices and circumstances. Identifying and focusing on common conditions, on high quality evidence, on organisational development, and on surveys of patient experience shows a clear and conscious bias towards both biomedicine and utilitarianism. Also, this move to a clinic-based, *disease*-focused service may lead to the GP, perhaps subconsciously, giving less priority to the circumstances of the particular patient than to the evidence for the disease. If this takes place, it represents a subtle but significant change in the GP's *situational appreciation*, orientating it away from the individual to an application of the evidence base to reach performance targets. Financially rewarding the achievement of target levels for process markers like cholesterol and blood pressure may compound this tendency. There is a clear risk here that we become, (or perhaps just as importantly, may *be seen* to become), a profession that treats patients as unwitting means to contractually driven ends. In philosophical terms, this defies Kant's 'formula of the end in itself', which demands that we treat 'humanity never simply as a means but always at the same time as an end'.[37] Also, as many of the quality indicators are based on process markers of chronic disease that we alter by using drugs, there is a risk that we become well-paid agents of a global pharmaceutical industry which increasingly drives the agenda of medical research.[26]

In choosing ten common clinical conditions for the QOF, there is a risk that other less common but serious conditions – multiple sclerosis, Parkinson's disease, rheumatoid arthritis for example, may receive less attention. There is also the fact that many patients, particularly the elderly, have co-morbidities. They suffer simultaneously from several different diseases – diabetes, hypertension, CHD – for example. Will they necessarily be best served by a system that focuses only on one aspect of their conditions at a time? There is still a requirement, under essential services, for practices to provide 'management of chronic disease in the manner determined by the practice, in discussion with the patient', but such management is not contractually monitored or directly rewarded.

Besides the management of other chronic diseases, essential services cover the care of patients who are ill or who perceive themselves to be ill, and the care of terminally ill patients. The first of these obviously deals with the traditional role of the GP, focused on the undifferentiated physical, psychological and social problems that patients bring. As discussed on page 21, these consultations often defy easy categorisation, requiring the full exercise of a GP's perceptual capacity, not just his or her biomedical knowledge. The lack of focus on less severe mental health problems is perhaps the most striking omission in the new contract. There are 41 QOF points (out of a total of 1050), for achieving targets in patients with severe long-term mental health problems, and no QOF points for dealing with less serious mental health problems, surely because it is very difficult to identify measurable criteria for assessing their management. Palliative and terminal care are hugely important and rewarding aspects of general practice, yet again, there are very few points to be achieved in this area.

The move to registration with a practice rather than a GP may serve to diminish continuity of care. This is important in achieving enablement[71] and in the development of the relationship between patient and doctor, and the confidence and trust gained thereby.

If we look at the contract in the light of Toon's 1994 analysis[4] discussed in pages 7–8, then we may be moving towards a model based more and more on anticipatory care and biomedicine, which provide measureable targets, and away from the teleological or hermeneutic models explored by Balint and McWhinney. The view that the nGMS contract, because it is measurement based, ignores some of the core values of general practice has been widely discussed.[72–74] Although it may be reasonably claimed that we need hard data to justify the increasing amounts spent in primary care in the NHS, I argue below that there are ways of measuring in general practice, which reflect to some degree the Balint/McWhinney tradition, which could be explored in future developments of the nGMS contract.

Hermeneutics and the Measurement of Enablement and Empathy

The six questions of the enablement instrument developed by Howie et al.[71] (see Appendix four) reflect the Balint/McWhinney tradition. Howie et al.[72] argue that 'the theory behind enablement is that adjustment and coping are important modifiers of outcome, and that "what is important in predicting outcome is how the respondent actually feels and perceives life"'.[75–76]

The enablement score, based on whether a doctor helps a patient understand his or her illness, and thereby is enabled to cope with both the illness and life (questions 1–3) is essentially hermeneutic. The further three questions on whether the doctor has helped the patient to keep him or herself healthy, be confident about his or her health and to be able to help him or herself, imply a teleology based on good health (correctly left undefined by the question and the GP), confidence and enablement.

Mercer's subsequent development and validation of the CARE (consultation and relational empathy) instrument, a patient questionnaire that measures the patient's perception of relational empathy in the consultation[66] could also be used within the context of the nGMS contract. It has recently been suggested that combining the CARE measure with Howie's CQI (which includes enablement, consultation length, and 'knowing the doctor well') may provide a composite measure (see Appendix five), which more fully reflects the doctor's inter–personal effectiveness than current nGMS measures.[68]

Ethics, Measurement and Accountability

There is a wider ethical concern here, however, about measurement and the nGMS contract. This use of measurement in public services is an important issue, not just for general practice, but also for contemporary society as a whole. In the third of her 2002 Reith lectures[77] on public accountability, the philosopher Onora O'Neill stated:

> *the real focus is on performance indicators chosen for ease of measurement and control rather than because they measure quality of performance accurately. Most people working in the public service have a reasonable sense not only of the specific clinical, educational, policing or other goals for which they work, but also of central ethical standards that they must meet. They know that these complex sets of goals may have to be relegated if they are required to run in a race to improve performance indicators. Even these who devise the indicators know that they are at very best surrogates for the real objectives.*

O'Neill's cautionary words should alert us to the dangers of attempting to measure complex behaviours, interactions and outcomes in general practice by using numerically based performance indicators.

It is in this area that the practical reasoning approach explored in this paper shows its strength, not just in dealing with patient–doctor interactions, but in a much wider sense, and specifically in responding to the this new contract. On pages 14–15, I discussed the need to respond correctly to new situations for which previous rules and principles may leave us unprepared. Perceptual capacity enables precisely this – an alert, questioning, sceptical but reasoned responsiveness to these new circumstances. It applies in responding to a new contract as much as in the consultation, and enables us to make correct decisions for our patients at an organisational as well as an individual patient level. Echoing the epigraph to this section, I suggest that measurement-based scientific knowledge is necessary, but quite insufficient, to achieve this on its own.

Conclusion

The discussion above draws heavily on McWhinney's thinking.[5] His clearly expressed ideas are of a discipline based on the relationship between the doctor and the patient, on individuals rather than diseases, and on an organismic view of the body and a rejection of mind–body duality.

I have set out a discussion of a modern conception of Aristotelian *phronesis* or practical reasoning in general practice, which I describe as *the practice of perception*. The aspects discussed – a grasp of the priority of the particular, and situational appreciation, which includes the appropriate use of imagination and the emotions – seem to me to fit together in a way that enables the GP to acknowledge and understand the complicated business of 'sorting the unsorted'. It enables us to negotiate uncertainty and complexity, while acknowledging their existence and importance.

I have quoted Aristotle in the epigraph to this chapter.[NE1104a5-10] Doctors and navigators may use representations of reality in the form of charts or clinical guidelines, but must choose a course based on all the hard realities of where they actually are, that place in the world where our decisions have to be made.

The practice of perception, by allowing the inclusion in deliberation of *all* important aspects impinging on a situation, also acknowledges that some problems may be, in medical terms, unsortable, and may have to be sorted outside the medical paradigm of the day, but within the terms of a relationship between two individual human beings who happen, on that day, in that situation, to be a doctor and a patient. This is important in resisting the increasing medicalisation of life (see footnote vi, p.7). Judgement in general practice is not only judgement of medical matters, but also judgement of what is medical and what is not.

At the root of the approach is a degree of subjectivity. A good GP is someone who is able, *because of who he or she is, and what he or she does*, to 'get things right', to paraphrase Wiggins.[10, pp.236-37] The making of a judgement contains elements of subjectivity. Judgements are always open to challenge, debate and discussion. What we can *aim for*, however,[NE1141b13-14] is attaining the best than can be achieved for that patient in that situation, through *the practice of perception*. The assessment of the video component of the MRCGP examination seems, reassuringly, to be a measure of perceptual capacity. The nGMS contract offers challenges to some of the core values of general practice, including a lack of focus on the individual patient and on the perceptual capacity of the doctor. There is no doubt, however, that it will evolve, and may benefit from the inclusion of an instrument that reflects the hermeneutic tradition of general practice.[68]

Although the discussion has centred on general practice, I believe that the approach is also appropriate for medicine in general, as suggested by Leder[53] and Hunter.[54] I suggest that if we were to adopt such an approach, we might avoid the over-simplified objectivity of medicine today, and become a profession that understands itself and its patients better than we currently do.

Appendix One
Dr Lawrence's Problem

Margaret Smith is seventy-nine years old and has been widowed for ten years. She lives alone on the third floor of a block of council flats without a lift, in a large city. Her son, Mark, is an alcoholic who lives nearby. He is frequently in trouble with the police and borrows money from her, which he never returns. Her daughter emigrated to Australia many years ago, largely because her father, now dead, was frequently violent to her and her mother. She is not in touch with her mother. Mrs Smith has two grandchildren in Australia whom she has never seen. Some of her neighbours take drugs, and she is often afraid to go out.

Her GP of ten years, Dr John Lawrence, is a well-respected, experienced and conscientious doctor. He is concerned about Mrs Smith, who has recently developed breast cancer. She has had surgery and has been advised by the hospital to have chemotherapy and radiotherapy. However, she is unsure about having further treatment. She says that she now feels pretty well, but also that she doesn't really care how long she lives. She suffers from arthritis of the hips, high blood pressure and diabetes, but doesn't take her tablets regularly, and her blood tests and blood pressure reflect very poor control. Dr Lawrence has spent a great deal of time listening to her concerns. He has told his patient that more chemotherapy may well extend her life, but that it will last six months, and will make her feel unwell while she is having it. Radiotherapy, in contrast, will last one month, carries fewer side-effects, and would decrease her chance of local recurrence by twenty per cent. He encouraged her to consider this. Mrs Smith, after much discussion, eventually decides to have no further treatment, and wants, as she puts it, 'to take her chances'.

The health visitor has been critical of Dr Lawrence's management, suggesting that he should be doing more to persuade Mrs Smith to accept treatment. She has also suggested that Mrs Smith should be offered anti-depressant medication.

Dr Lawrence's elderly mother recently died after treatment for breast cancer.

Practising Perception

There are well-defined evidence-based guidelines for the management of some of Mrs Smith's illnesses: breast cancer, diabetes and hypertension (see: www.sign.ac.uk). Dr Lawrence is well aware of them and has discussed some of them with Mrs Smith. As a conscientious GP, he has also read about the four principles approach to medical ethics (see page 23). In this context, he is unsure how helpful they are. He is keen not to harm his patient (non-maleficence) and is worried that chemotherapy and radiotherapy will do precisely this, in the short term. At the same time, pursuing those treatments *may* extend her life – a beneficent effect. He certainly wishes to respect his patient's autonomous decision. The issue of justice does not seem immediately relevant, in these circumstances.

Dr Lawrence's judgement is that she does not have a depressive illness, but is sad because of the circumstances of her long and difficult life. He has listened at length to Mrs Smith's story, not just of her illness, but of her family life and current social problems. Her housing and the sadness associated with her children cannot be remedied medically. However, Mrs Smith much appreciates the time that Dr Lawrence spends with her, allowing her to talk about concerns and her family situation.

Dr Lawrence, because of his mother's recent death from breast cancer, has an enhanced degree of emotional engagement with the situation. He is able to imagine, from his mother's own experience, how both the disease and further treatment may affect his patient in the future. He has allowed her to express her fears and concerns about the future, and responds appropriately by explaining what may happen to her. He has also organised a significant event analysis at the practice on the situation, thus involving the health visitor who expressed divergent views.

The way that Dr Lawrence has managed this case demonstrates well *the practice of perception*. He looks at the particular situation, and applies to it his capacity, born of much experience, for 'situational appreciation'. He considers the medical evidence on how his patient may be managed, as well as, rather obliquely, the four principles approach. However, his deliberative specification also takes into account many other non-medical aspects of the situation – his patient's own directly and obliquely expressed views, and her difficult social and family circumstances. He imagines how Mrs Smith's disease may affect her, and then uses his emotional experience as a bereaved son to respond in a way that aims to achieve what is best for this patient. At the same time, he avoids over-engagement, which may be detrimental both to him and Mrs Smith.

Finally, he uses the experience of disagreement between himself and another health professional to explore the situation at a significant event analysis, allowing free discussion of issues. This will allow both the health visitor and himself to reflect on their experience of this patient, and may improve both his judgement and that of others in the future.

Appendix Two

Criteria for video assessment of consultations submitted to the National Office for Summative Assessment.

	CRITERIA
ERROR/S	· The presence of a single major error on the consultation or of a number of minor errors should lead to consideration of referral · serious error = causes actual/potential harm · minor error = inconvenience only
LISTENING	· Identify and elucidate reasons for attendance · A credible/acceptable plan should be negotiated
ACTION	· Appropriate action to identify patient's problems · Reasonable investigations/referrals · Help sought when necessary · Patient's problem should be managed appropriately
UNDERSTANDING	· GP registrar understands process/outcome of consultation · Actions explained · Obvious shortcomings identified and relevant background mentioned

RATING SCALE

1 Refer
2 Probably Refer
3 Bare Pass
4 Competent
5 Good
6 Excellent

OVERALL ASSESSMENT

R+ Clear Refer
R Refer
P Pass
P+ Clear Pass

From: website of the National Office for Summative Assessment: www.nosa.org.uk

Appendix Three
Criteria for Video Assessment of Consulting Skills for the MRCGP Examination

DISCOVER THE REASONS FOR THE PATIENT'S ATTENDANCE

a. ELICIT AN ACCOUNT OF THE SYMPTOM(S)

(P) PC1: the doctor is seen to encourage the patient's contribution at appropriate points in the consultation

(M) PC2: the doctor is seen to respond to signals (cues) that lead to a deeper understanding of the problem

b. OBTAIN RELEVANT ITEMS OF SOCIAL AND OCCUPATIONAL CIRCUMSTANCES

(P) PC3: the doctor uses appropriate psychological and social information to place the complaint(s) in context

c. EXPLORE THE PATIENT'S HEALTH UNDERSTANDING

(P) PC4: the doctor explores the patient's health understanding

DEFINE THE CLINICAL PROBLEM(S)

a. OBTAIN ADDITIONAL INFORMATION ABOUT THE SYMPTOMS, AND OTHER DETAILS OF MEDICAL HISTORY

(P) PC5: the doctor obtains sufficient information to include or exclude likely relevant significant conditions

b. ASSESS THE PATIENT BY APPROPRIATE PHYSICAL AND MENTAL EXAMINATION

(P) PC6: the physical/mental examination chosen is likely to confirm or disprove hypotheses that could reasonably have been formed OR is designed to address a patient's concern

c. MAKE A WORKING DIAGNOSIS

(P) PC7: the doctor appears to make a clinically appropriate working diagnosis

EXPLAIN THE PROBLEM(S) TO THE PATIENT

a. SHARE THE FINDINGS WITH THE PATIENT

(P) PC8: the doctor explains the problem or diagnosis in appropriate language

(M) PC9: the doctor's explanation incorporates some or all of the patient's health beliefs

b. ENSURE THAT THE EXPLANATION IS UNDERSTOOD AND ACCEPTED BY THE PATIENT

(M) PC10: the doctor specifically seeks to confirm the patient's understanding of the diagnosis

ADDRESS THE PATIENT'S PROBLEM(S)

a. CHOOSE AN APPROPRIATE FORM OF MANAGEMENT

(P) PC11: the management plan (including any prescription) is appropriate for the working diagnosis, reflecting a good understanding of modern accepted medical practice

b. INVOLVE THE PATIENT IN THE MANAGEMENT PLAN

(P) PC12: the patient is given the opportunity to be involved in significant management decisions

MAKE EFFECTIVE USE OF THE CONSULTATION

a. MAKE EFFECTIVE USE OF RESOURCES

(M) PC13: in prescribing the doctor takes steps to enhance concordance, by exploring and responding to the patient's understanding of the treatment

(P) PC14: the doctor specifies the conditions and interval for follow-up or review

(From: *Video assessment of consulting skills 2005: Workbook and instructions.* Available at: www.rcgp.org.uk/exam/videoworkbook/intro.asp?menuid=76)

Appendix Four
Enablement Instrument

CONSULTATION QUALITY INDEX

PLEASE COMPLETE THE QUESTIONS BELOW AFTER YOU HAVE SEEN THE DOCTOR.

1) As a result of your visit to the doctor today, do you feel you are... *(please tick one box in each row)*:-

	MUCH BETTER	BETTER	SAME OR LESS	NOT APPLICABLE
able to cope with life	☐	☐	☐	☐
able to understand your illness	☐	☐	☐	☐
able to cope with your illness	☐	☐	☐	☐
able to keep yourself healthy	☐	☐	☐	☐

	MUCH MORE	MORE	SAME OR LESS	NOT APPLICABLE
confident about your health	☐	☐	☐	☐
able to help yourself	☐	☐	☐	☐

From: Howie J, Heaney D, Maxwell M, Walker J, *et al*. Quality at general practice consultations: cross sectional survey. *British Medical Journal* 1999: **319**; 738-743. Reproduced with permission from the BMJ Publishing Group.

Appendix Five
New Consultation Quality Index

PLEASE COMPLETE THE QUESTIONS BELOW AFTER YOU HAVE SEEN THE DOCTOR.

1) As a result of your visit to the doctor today, do you feel you are... *(please tick one box in each row)*:-

	MUCH BETTER	BETTER	SAME OR LESS	NOT APPLICABLE
able to cope with life	☐	☐	☐	☐
able to understand your illness	☐	☐	☐	☐
able to cope with your illness	☐	☐	☐	☐
able to keep yourself healthy	☐	☐	☐	☐

	MUCH MORE	MORE	SAME OR LESS	NOT APPLICABLE
confident about your health	☐	☐	☐	☐
able to help yourself	☐	☐	☐	☐

2) What language(s) - other than English - do you routinely speak at home?

3) If your consultation with the doctor used a language other than English, please write down the language you used:-

4) How well do you know the doctor you saw today? *(please place a circle round one of the numbers below)*:-

(don't know doctor at all) 1 2 3 4 5 *(know doctor very well)*

FOR DOCTOR'S USE ONLY:

GP ID: _____ DATE: _____

START TIME: _____ END TIME: _____

Please rate the following statements about today's consultation. Please tick one box for each statement and **answer every statement**.

How was the doctor at . . .	Poor	Fair	Good	Very Good	Excellent	Does Not Apply
1. Making you feel at ease . . . *(being friendly and warm towards you, treating you with respect; not cold or abrupt)*	☐	☐	☐	☐	☐	☐
2. Letting you tell your 'story' . . . *(giving you time to fully describe your illness in your own words; not interrupting or diverting you)*	☐	☐	☐	☐	☐	☐
3. Really listening . . . *(paying close attention to what you were saying; not looking at the notes or computer as you were talking)*	☐	☐	☐	☐	☐	☐
4. Being interested in you as a whole person . . . *(asking/knowing relevant details about your life, your situation; not treating you as 'just a number')*	☐	☐	☐	☐	☐	☐
5. Fully understanding your concerns . . . *(communicating that he/she had accurately understood your concerns; not overlooking or dismissing anything)*	☐	☐	☐	☐	☐	☐
6. Showing care and compassion . . . *(seeming genuinely concerned, connecting with you on a human level; not being indifferent or 'detached')*	☐	☐	☐	☐	☐	☐
7. Being Positive . . . *(having a positive approach and a positive attitude; being honest but not negative about your problems)*	☐	☐	☐	☐	☐	☐
8. Explaining things clearly . . . *(fully answering your questions, explaining clearly, giving you adequate information; not being vague*	☐	☐	☐	☐	☐	☐
9. Helping you to take control . . . *(exploring with you what you can do to improve your health yourself; encouraging rather than "lecturing" you)*	☐	☐	☐	☐	☐	☐
10. Making a plan of action with you . . . *(discussing the options, involving you in decisions as much as you want to be involved; not ignoring your views)*	☐	☐	☐	☐	☐	☐

5) Please tick here if someone helped you to complete this questionnaire:- ☐

Adapted from: Mercer S, Reynolds W. Empathy and quality of care. *Br J Gen Pract* 2002; **52:** S9–S12. (Quality supplement)
(Discussed in reference 68: Howie J, Heaney D, Maxwell M, Freeman, G, Mercer S. Performance indicator scoring (letter). *Br J Gen Pract* 2004, **54;** 624)

References

All references to Aristotle's *Nicomachean Ethics* are in the generally used form: NE1107b1-4. Except where indicated, translations of the *Nicomachean Ethics* are those of Ross.[41]

1. Holt T. (Ed.) *Complexity for clinicians.* Oxford: Radcliffe Publishing, 2004.
2. Plsek P, Greenhalgh T. The challenge of complexity in health care. *BMJ* 2001; **323**: 625–28.
3. Wilson T, Holt T, Greenhalgh T. Complexity and Clinical Care. *BMJ* 2001; **323**: 685–88.
4. Toon P. *Occasional Paper No 65. What is Good General Practice?* London: Royal College of General Practitioners, 1994.
5. McWhinney I. The Pickles lecture: the importance of being different. *Br J Gen Pract* 1996; **46**: 433–36.
6. Wiggins D. A Sensible Subjectivism. In: Wiggins D. *Needs, Value Truth* (third edition). Oxford: Clarendon Press, 2002; pp.185–214.
7. McDowell J. Virtue and Reason. In: McDowell J. *Mind, Value and Reality.* Cambridge: Harvard University Press, 1998; pp.50–73.
8. Nussbaum M. The Discernment of Perception: An Aristotelian Conception of Private and Public Rationality. In: Sherman N (ed). *Aristotle's Ethics: Critical Essays.* Lanham: Rowman and Littlefield Publishers Inc, 1999; pp.145–81.
9. Purves I. The Changing Consultation. In: Harrison J and van Zwanenberg T (eds). *GP Tomorrow.* Oxford: Radcliffe Medical Press, 2002; pp.33–47.
10. Wiggins D. Deliberation and Practical Reason. In: Wiggins D. *Needs, Value Truth* (third edition). Oxford: Clarendon Press, 2002; pp.215–37.
11. Beauchamp T and Childress J. *Principles of Medical Ethics* (fifth edition). Oxford: Oxford University Press, 2001.
12. Greenhalgh T. Intuition and evidence – uneasy bedfellows? *Br J Gen Pract* 2002; **52**: 395–400.
13. Collings J. General Practice in England Today. *Lancet* 1950; March 25th: 555–85.
14. Spence J. *The Purpose and Practice of Medicine.* Oxford: Oxford University Press, 1960.
15. Fry J. *Common Diseases; their nature, incidence and care.* Lancaster: MTP Press, 1985.
16. Tudor Hart J. *A New Kind of Doctor.* London: Merlin Press, 1988.
17. Balint M. *The Doctor, his Patient and the Illness.* London: Pitman Medical, 1964.
18. Royal College of General Practitioners. *What sort of doctor?* London: RCGP, 1985.
19. General Medical Council. *Good Medical Practice.* London: General Medical Council, 2001.
20. Sheehan M. Health Care and (a kind of) virtue ethics. In: Hayry M, Takala T and Herissone-Kelly P (eds). *Bioethics and Social Reality.* Amsterdam/New York: Rodopi, 2005.
21. Popper K. *Conjectures and Refutations: The Growth of Scientific Knowledge* (fifth edition 1989, revised). London: Routledge and Kegan Paul, 1963.
22. McWhinney I. *A Textbook of Family Medicine.* New York/Oxford: Oxford University Press, 1989.
23. Power M. *The Audit Society: rituals of verification.* Oxford: Oxford University Press, 1997.
24. Martin R. NHS waiting lists and evidence of national or local failure: analysis of health service data. *BMJ* 2003; **326**: 188–92.
25. Le Fanu J. *The Rise and Fall of Modern Medicine.* London: Little, Brown and Company (UK), 1999.
26. Bodenheimer T. Uneasy Alliance – clinical investigators and the pharmaceutical industry. *New Eng J Med* 2000; **342**: 1539–44.
27. Moynihan R. The making of a disease: female sexual dysfunction. *BMJ* 2003; **326**: 45–47.
28. Nussbaum M. *Aristotle's De Motu Animalium.* Princeton: Princeton University Press, 1978.
29. Toon P. *Occasional Paper No. 78. Towards a Philosophy of General Practice: a Study of the Virtuous Practitioner.* London: Royal College of General Practitioners, 1999.
30. McIntyre A. *After Virtue: a study in moral theory* (second edition). London: Duckworth, 1985.
31. Sackett D, Rosenberg W, Muir Gray J, Haynes B *et al.* Evidence-based medicine: what it is and what it isn't. *BMJ* 1996; **312**: 71–72.
32. Greenhalgh T, Hurwitz B (eds). *Narrative Based Medicine.* London: BMJ Books, 1998.
33. Greenhalgh T. Narrative based medicine in an evidence based world. In: Greenhalgh T and Hurwitz B (eds). *Narrative Based Medicine.* London: BMJ Books, 1998; pp.247–66.
34. Foss L. *The end of modern medicine: biomedical medicine under a microscope.* New York: State University of New York Press, 2002.
35. Harrington A. *Reenchanted science: holism in German culture from Wilhelm II to Hitler.* Princeton: Princeton University Press, 1996.
36. Barnes B. Thomas Kuhn. In: Skinner Q (ed). *The Return of Grand Theory in the Human Sciences.* Cambridge: Cambridge University Press, 1985.
37. O'Neill O. Kantian Ethics. In: Singer P (ed). *A Companion to Ethics.* Oxford: Blackwell Reference, 1993; pp.175–85.
38. Pettit P. Consequentialism. In: Singer P (ed). *A Companion to Ethics.* Oxford: Blackwell Reference, 1993; pp.230–41.
39. Wittgenstein, L. *Philosophical Investigations.* (translated by Anscombe, G, third edition, Oxford: Blackwell Publishers, 2001.
40. Carritt E. *The Theory of Morals: an Introduction to Ethical Philosophy,* London: Oxford University Press, 1928.
41. Ross D. (translator) *Aristotle: The Nicomachean Ethics.* Oxford: Oxford University Press. (Oxford

41. (...World's Classics edition 1953, revised Ackrill J, Urmson J. 1988).
42. Blackburn S. *A Dictionary of Philosophy.* Oxford: Oxford University Press, 1994.
43. Ubel P. *Pricing Life; Why It's Time for Health Care Rationing.* Cambridge, Massachusetts: MIT Press, 2000.
44. Williams, B. A Critique of Utilitarianism. In: Cahn S and Markie P (eds). *Ethics: history, theory and contemporary themes.* Oxford: Oxford University Press, 1998; pp.566–83.
45. Wiggins D. Truth, Invention and the Meaning of Life. In: Wiggins D. *Needs, Value, Truth* (third edition). Oxford: Clarendon Press, 2002; pp.87–137.
46. Irwin T. *Aristotle: Nicomachean Ethics (second edition)*, Indianapolis/Cambridge: Hackett Publishing Company Inc, 1999.
47. Scottish Intercollegiate Guidelines Network. Available at: www.sign.ac.uk.
48. Brunschwig J, Lloyd G (eds). *Greek Thought: A Guide to Classical Knowledge.* Cambridge: The Belknap Press of Harvard University Press, 2000.
49. Rogers W. Are Guidelines ethical? Some considerations for general practice. *Br J Gen Pract* 2002; **52**: 663–68.
50. Blackburn S. *Ruling Passions.* Oxford: Oxford University Press, 1998.
51. *Chambers Dictionary.* Edinburgh: W&R Chambers Ltd, 1972.
52. Gould SJ. The median isn't the message. In: Greenhalgh T and Hurwitz B (eds). *Narrative Based Medicine.* London: BMJ Books, 1998.
53. Leder D. Clinical Interpretation: the hermeneutics of medicine. *Theoretical Medicine* 1990; **11**: 9–24.
54. Hunter KM. Narrative, Literature, and the Clinical Exercise of Practical Reason. *J Med Philos* 1996; **21**: 303–20.
55. Schon D. *The Reflective Practitioner: how professionals think in action.* Aldershot: Ashgate/Arena Press, 1991.
56. Dreyfus H, Dreyfus S. *Mind over Machine: the Power of Human Intuition and Expertise in the Era of the Computer.* Oxford: Basil Blackwell, 1986.
57. Macnaughton J. Arts and Humanities in Medical Education. In: Harrison J and van Zwanenberg T (eds). *GP Tomorrow.* Oxford: Radcliffe Medical Press, 2002; pp.67–77.
58. Kirwan M, Armstrong D. Investigation into burnout in a sample of British general practitioners. *Br J Gen Pract* 1995; **45**: 259–60.
59. Gomori G, Atlas J (eds). *Attila Jozsef: Selected poems and texts* (translated from the Hungarian by John Bakti). Cheadle: Carcanet Press, 1973.
60. www.globalfamilydoctor.com (An oration given by Professor Ian McWhinney at the WONCA Europe conference, Vienna, 2000.)
61. www.nosa.org.uk
62. www.rcgp.org.uk/exam/regulations/regu.asp?menuid=76
63. Neighbour R. *The Inner Consultation.* Newbury: Petroc Press, 1987.
64. Mercer S, Reynolds W. Empathy and Quality of Care. *Br J Gen Pract* 2002; **52**: S9–S12.
65. Morse J, Anderson G, Botter J *et al.* Exploring empathy: a conceptual fit for nursing practice? *Image J Nurs Sch* 1992; **24**: 273–80.
66. Mercer S, Maxwell M, Heaney D, Watt G. The consultation and relational empathy (CARE) measure: development of an empathy-based consultation process measure. *Fam Pract* 2004; **21**: 699–705.
67. Marshall M, Roland M. The new contract: renaissance or requiem for general practice. [editorial] *Br J Gen Pract* 2002; **52**: 205–06.
68. Howie J, Heaney D, Maxwell M, Freeman, G, Mercer S. Performance indicator scoring. [letter] *Br J Gen Pract* 2004; **54**: 624.
69. NHS Confederation/British Medical Association. New GMS Contract 2003; investing in general practice. London: BMA Publishing, 2003.
70. NHS Confederation/British Medical Association. New GMS Contract 2003; investing in general practice. Supporting documentation. London: BMA Publishing, 2003.
71. Howie J, Heaney D, Maxwell M, Walker J, *et al.* Quality at general practice consultations: cross sectional survey. *BMJ* 1999; **319**: 738–43.
72. Howie J, Heaney D, Maxwell M. Quality, core values and the general practice consultation: issues of definition, measurement and delivery. *Fam Pract* 2004; **21**: 458–68.
73. Heath I. The cawing of the crow . . . *Br J Gen Pract* 2004; **54**: 320–21.
74. Gillies J. What is medicine for? [Editorial] *Update.* 2002; 31st October: 336.
75. Lazarus RS. *Patterns of Adjustment,* New York: McGraw-Hill, 1976.
76. Cox T. *Stress.* London: McMillan, 1981.
77. O'Neill O. *A question of trust: the BBC Reith Lectures* Cambridge: Cambridge University Press. 2002; pp.54–55.